Chapter 1

What this book is and what it isn't

Since the first edition of this ebook was published, the business of diagnosing and treating sleep apnea has been evolving rapidly as the home sleep testing (HST) gains popularity. The in-laboratory, attended sleep test, called a polysomnogram, is still considered the "gold standard" for sleep testing but the number of people who have sleep apnea makes it impractical for all of them to be evaluated in a full sleep disorders center, or even in a specialty sleep related breathing disorder lab.

The resulting increased usage of HST, sometimes coupled with even less support in adapting to CPAP therapy by the medical equipment provider because of insurance reimbursement, may make this ebook even more useful for the new CPAP user. I have also developed an online, video based program covering this information. Please see: www.practicalhealthstrategies.com and follow the "Online Programs" link to the "Self-Directed Programs" link. The video program is free and I encourage you to also view the videos. In my opinion, CPAP machines should be available "over the counter" without prescription, once there are evidence based guidelines for setting the pressure, which will make monographs such as this, and the related videos, more useful.

In this book I am going to share some of my knowledge dealing with most of the problems people have getting used to sleeping with their CPAP machine and mask. This book is targeted toward the BEGINNER CPAP user. It is not a medical textbook nor is it a technical book.

This book will make you more knowledgeable about your sleep apnea and about your CPAP machine. There are no guarantees in life, but this book should give you the information you need to solve many of your problems with your CPAP machine and mask. For the problems you can't solve yourself, it will give you the information you need to better communicate with your doctor, the sleep lab, and the therapist or technologist from the medical equipment supplier. If you have a persistent problem with your CPAP you probably need more specific guidance and I encourage you to talk with your local professionals. I hope this book will expedite that discussion solution.

I have almost thirty years of experience in sleep disorders and their treatments, across the range of sleep disorders and sleep apnea has been prominent. Every day I have dealt with people's problems with their CPAP machines. I regularly conduct sleep disorders and CPAP support group meetings.

However, this book does **NOT** give medical advice. Only YOUR doctor can give you medical advice. All professional advice, be it legal, financial, medical, psychological or otherwise, requires one-on-one communication with the professional and cannot be provided in a book or other publication. Personally, I believe this one-on-one communication should also be face-to-face in the case of medical advice.

Also, it is my experience that many people leave the doctor's office with a misunderstanding about their sleep apnea, not because the doctor didn't do a good job of explaining, but because the doctor gave them so much information it was overwhelming.

We are going to first talk about sleep apnea because only by understanding what apnea is, and how it does its harm, can you understand what you are trying to accomplish with your therapy.

We are also going to discuss some of the alternative therapies for sleep apnea and what factors might make you a candidate for one of them. I will share with you why CPAP is so often the prescribed treatment and why your doctor seems to prefer CPAP over other therapies.

There is a lot of free information available about sleep apnea and CPAP usage. For the most part this information is not incorrect, but it is often incomplete or biased. In this book I will present a complete, and relatively unbiased, overview of sleep apnea and how to adjust to living with CPAP.

I do, however, have one bias: CPAP can be one of the most cost effective therapies in modern medicine but it will do you no good if you do not use it. So I believe there should be as much emphasis on using it as there is on ordering it in the first place.

It often takes effort and patience to acclimate to the machine and mask. The goal of this book is to help.

I avoid unscientific explanations and unsubstantiated or irrational therapies. My goal has been to write to an intelligent reader who may not have specialized medical knowledge.

First we'll discuss sleep apnea, how it is diagnosed, how it does its damage and why it is bad for you, the problems commonly encountered adapting to CPAP therapy, and what you can do about them. This section should help you understand your sleep disorder and help you better communicate with your doctor.

Then there is a question and answer section. This section covers information that just didn't fit well into the narrative format and sometimes overlaps with the previous section.

Next, there is a glossary. This section can also be a very good source for specific information and understanding. I have tried to include all specific terminology used in the book.

Finally, there are several appendices.

The first gives some helpful hints for obtaining quality sleep. The second is a questionnaire we sometimes use to help people decide if they might need to be evaluated for sleep apnea. The third is a form we use to give patients the results of their sleep studies. The two forms are image files and may be hard to view on your ereader. The fourth tells you a little about me.

The sleep disorders field continues to evolve.

Please visit my website www.practicalhealthstrategies.com, please connect with us on Facebook, Google+, LinkedIn and/or Twitter. Online programs are available and "Health Updates" offer random updates on relevant published research.

Chapter 2

What is sleep apnea?

The word "apnea" means to not breathe, or to stop breathing, and the expression "sleep apnea" means to stop breathing in your sleep.

By definition, in the sleep disorders field, we do not count an apnea unless it is at least ten seconds in duration, but it can be significantly longer. For most people the **average** apnea is somewhere between about 15 and about 30 seconds or so. But, this can vary greatly.

> Of course, there has to be a specific and technical definition of apnea so that we are all talking about the same thing. We begin measuring an event when the airflow decreases by 90% or more of the baseline breathing prior to the event. That means there may be a residual airflow of up to 10%. That amount of airflow is considered insufficient to supply your physiological needs (supplying oxygen and removing carbon dioxide) and is merely flushing the "dead space" the parts of your ventilator structures that do not exchange respiratory gases. (We use two different airflow sensors in the sleep lab utilizing two different technologies to be sure we can detect small decreases in airflow while still detecting very small amounts of residual airflow.) The event must last for at least ten seconds, as mentioned.

The diagnosis of sleep apnea as a sleep disorder refers to stopping breathing repeatedly during the night.

The severity of your apnea....

To be diagnosed with sleep apnea, the definition specifies that an adult must stop breathing five or more times per hour of sleep. (There is a different definition in children which requires only one per hour.) One of the shortcomings of the home sleep tests is that most of them do not actually record the brainwaves (EEG) to be able to document the actual amount of sleep time. They may, therefore, either over or under estimate the amount of sleep apnea.

Sleep apnea is classified as mild, moderate or severe based on how frequently you stop breathing.

> Mild: 5 up to 15 times per hour of sleep
> Moderate: 15 up to 30 times per hour of sleep
> Severe: 30 or more times per hour

"Wouldn't I know it if I stopped breathing?" you ask.

The simple answer is: "Usually not, but sometimes."

So, what happens when you stop breathing in your sleep?

This is a somewhat complicated and involved question which we will get more into later. But for now, the immediate effect is that it disturbs your sleep making it less restful.

In the long term, however, sleep apnea has serious implications for your health. Let's take a minute and talk about the apnea itself.

In the sleep lab, we classify each and every time you stop breathing as one of three types of apnea. In the case of home sleep tests, it depends upon the specific model of HST instrument used as to whether the classification can be made but most do.

Although the relative percentage of each type is of interest to your sleep doctor, it usually matters little to you, the apnea sufferer.

What kind of apnea do you have....

The three types of sleep apneic *events* are:

> Obstructive
> Central
> Mixed

Do not confuse "mixed" apnea, which refers to a specific type of respiratory *event*, with "complex" sleep apnea which refers to a type of sleep apnea *disorder*. I will explain later.

Obstructive sleep apnea is, by far, the most common type seen in the sleep disorders center and, if you are reading this book, is probably the type of sleep apnea you have been diagnosed.

Obstructive sleep apnea occurs when the upper airway collapses or "obstructs" as you try to breathe in. Thus the name. The collapse generally occurs as a collapse of the walls of the pharynx, an area you would typically refer to as your throat, but may also involve the soft palate and/or tongue falling back against the back of the pharynx.

Throughout this book, anytime "sleep apnea" is mentioned without further clarification, it is a safe assumption that we are referring to the obstructive variety.

> Think about it. In order to pull air through you nose or mouth and down into your lungs, you must create a negative pressure with your chest. If you pull too hard the airway can collapse, just like a straw in a milkshake. After the air flows through your nose, which is semi-rigid, it moves inside your skull, which is definitely rigid (my wife often reminds me of mine), as the nasal passages make their way to your throat. Below your throat, the trachea, popularly called the "windpipe", has rings of cartilage to keep it rigid. In between, in the area known as the pharynx, through which both food and air must pass, the tissue is soft. It is in this area that the airway can collapse.

Obstructive sleep apnea is far more than a mere "plumbing" problem, however. If it were just plumbing, then surgical correction and/or weight loss would have a very high success rate, which they don't. Among the contributing factors to obstructive sleep apnea are:

> Overweight/Obesity
> Facial structure and anomalies
> Tissue elasticity
> Sleep stage and/or position
> Respiratory control and/or respiratory muscle factors
> Nasal congestion and/or allergies
> Cardiac status

Obstructive sleep apnea syndrome is often abbreviated OSAS and refers to five or more obstructive events per hour of sleep. Sometimes it is referred to as obstructive sleep apnea/hypopnea syndrome because for most people some of their obstructive events are hypopneae, which I define for you in the next section.

Central sleep apnea occurs when you simply hold your breath in your sleep, not trying to breathe at all. There are several situations that can result in a central apnea, including simply no need to breathe at that time because you have sufficient oxygen, and not too much carbon dioxide, in your blood.

> We will discuss some of these causes of central sleep apnea later when we consider the problems you can have on your CPAP machine.

Central sleep apnea syndrome is abbreviated CSAS and refers to five or more central events per hour of sleep.

A mixed apnea is, as the name implies, partly central and partly obstructive. The definition of a mixed apnea is one that begins as a central apnea but becomes obstructive. At first you simply hold your breath but when you try to breathe the airway collapses and obstructs. A commonly seen pattern of repeated mixed apnea events, with periods of over-breathing (hyperventilation) in between, gives an excellent example of how defects in respiratory control can lead to the observed apnea and may provide insight into the natural history of all types of sleep apnea. (Sleep doctors use the expression "loop gain" when discussing this.)

At the present time, there is not a disorder called mixed sleep apnea syndrome as they are usually seen in patients with obstructive sleep apnea and account for a percentage of the events. The term mixed apnea refers, therefore, to the classification of an individual apnea. (Again, do not confuse this with "complex" apnea, described below.)

Other terms related to your apnea....

A few other terms you might hear in describing your sleep apnea include:

>Hypopnea (plural: hypopneae, technically correct, but usually just hypopneas)
>Complex sleep apnea
>Respiratory event
>Cheyne-Stokes respiration (CSR)
>Respiratory event related arousal (RERA)
>Upper airway resistance syndrome (UARS)
>Hypoventilation
>Sleep disordered breathing
>Desaturation, Saturation, "Sats", or "Desats"

Hypopnea has been called a "partial apnea" and occurs by the same mechanism as an obstructive apnea but the airflow is not completely blocked. As a practical matter, for our purposes a hypopnea can be considered the same as an apnea.

>Of course, there is a technical definition of hypopnea and, to confuse things more, there are actually two definitions which specify how much the airflow must be obstructed and how much the oxygen in the blood must decrease.

>One definition requires that the airflow decrease by at least 30% and the blood oxygen level must by at least 3% from the baseline level (recommended) and in the other definition the oxygen level must fall by at least 4% (acceptable). At the time of this writing, US Medicare does not recognize the "recommended" definition but does recognize the "acceptable" definition. The only requirement is that the same definition must be used throughout an entire study and it must be specified on the sleep study report. (These definitions have varied over the years which is why your older sleep study may not be accepted by the insurance company or Medicare.)

>Regardless, as a practical matter, moving too little air to supply your brain and your body with oxygen, and the associated sleep disruption, is essentially as bad as not moving any air. Your sleeping brain very quickly senses that your airflow is blocked,

whether completely or partially.

Complex sleep apnea is a combination of obstructive and central sleep apnea. Unlike a mixed apnea in which both central and obstructive characteristics occur in a single respiratory event (see below), complex sleep apnea occurs when some of the apneae are central and others are obstructive. Complex sleep apnea, therefore, refers to the classification of the patient's sleep apnea syndrome.

> As you might expect, there is a specific, technical definition of complex sleep apnea syndrome which specifies how many must be central and how many must be obstructive to consider it complex.

The expression "respiratory event" is often used generically to include any apnea (whether obstructive, mixed or central) or any hypopnea.

Cheyne-Stokes respiration, often abbreviated CSR, is a specific pattern of central apnea in which the airflow gradually diminishes until it stops and then gradually increases back to normal. CSR is a special case, often associated with heart failure, and we will not discuss it in depth. There are, however, specialized and rather expensive versions of positive airway pressure developed especially for CSR and for complex sleep apnea. (At the time of this writing, there is a scientific debate over the significance of CSR in heart failure.)

Sometimes, as the airway begins to collapse but before the airflow diminishes enough or the oxygen decreases enough to qualify as an apnea or hypopnea, the person will arouse enough from sleep to restore the airflow.   If this results in sleep related symptoms (such as unrestful sleep) the resulting sleep disturbance is referred to as "upper airway resistance syndrome" or UARS and, although most of the data on UARS relates to the resulting sleep disturbance, there is probably an effect on your blood pressure and heart as with sleep apnea.

The sleep disturbances or brain wave "arousals" associated with respiratory events, or near events as in UARS, are sometimes referred to as "respiratory event related arousals" or RERAs. A RERA can only be determined if there are EEG, brainwave, electrodes used in the study.

> Sometimes these arousals may result in a leg jerk that might be counted as a "periodic limb movement". When this occurs on the night of the CPAP trial, it has been called "CPAP kick" and probably needs no further treatment. Of course, the fact that some periodic leg jerks are an artifact of the sleep apnea and its treatment, does not mean that primary periodic limb movements cannot also coexist with sleep apnea. The current International Classification of Sleep Disorders requires that leg jerks must be associated with symptoms, not just an observation on the sleep study, to qualify as a diagnosis.

Hypoventilation refers to shallow breathing, so shallow as to result in accumulation of carbon dioxide in the bloodstream, and often also to a lower than normal level of oxygen. The most common cause of this in the sleep lab setting is obesity but there are other causes such as scoliosis. Of course, hypoventilation can coexist with sleep apnea, of any type.

All of the various types of sleep apnea, as well as RERAs and UARS, snoring, and hypoventilation are collectively referred to as "sleep disordered breathing" or SDB.

During a sleep study, the oxygen level in the blood is monitored using an instrument called a "pulse oximeter" which uses a light beam to determine what percentage of the total oxygen carrying capacity of the blood is actually carrying oxygen.

> Blood cells with oxygen attached are bright red. Blood cells without oxygen are dark red. Using a light, red filters, and photocells, the oximeter measures the amount of bright red and dark red light that is transmitted through your finger. By comparing these, it can calculate the ratio and calculate what percentage is carrying oxygen.

This is referred to as the "saturation" or "sat" of the blood's oxygen carrying capacity. It is expressed as a percentage and, in a normal, healthy individual will be in the 96 to 98 percent range. It should not be confused with an arterial blood gas, ABG, which may have similar values if you are at sea level.

> The pulse oximeter is unable to measure absolute oxygen levels so, for example, if you are very anemic you might have an acceptable oxygen saturation level but still have too little oxygen in your blood in an absolute sense.

> Carbon monoxide makes red blood cells bright red but the cells are unable to carry oxygen and the carbon monoxide attaches more strongly and longer to the blood cell longer than the oxygen. Because of this, the oximeter is inaccurate in the presence of carbon monoxide. This is most important in the sleep lab because the oximeters can read inaccurately high for smokers.

When the oxygen saturation falls during a respiratory event, it is referred to as a "desaturation" or "desat" and is expressed as the number of percentage points it falls. Thus, if the saturation is 96% while you are breathing and drops to 90% due to an apnea, the desaturation, or desat, is six percentage points, but may be stated as "six percent" (even though that is not exactly correct in a mathematical sense).

> In the case of a normal baseline of 96 to 98 percent this difference can be insignificant. In fact, so insignificant that the current scoring manual ignores the distinction. In the case of a very low baseline saturation, this can be a measurable difference.

How much you will desat with a particular respiratory event is a complex multifactorial function but, in general, severely obese individuals and people with lung disease, such as COPD, will desaturate more. Conversely, a young, relatively healthy, mildly overweight adult might desaturate very little even with many respiratory events.

Also, contrary to what you might at first think, your lowest saturation of the night might not correlate with your longest respiratory event of the night. And the desaturation associated with apnea may not be lower than the desaturation associated with a hypopnea, regardless of their relative lengths.

Chapter 3

What are some of the Health effects of sleep apnea?

As we alluded to earlier, the consequences of having sleep apnea can be divided into short and moderate time frame and longer time frame effects, however, for this discussion we will talk about those effects caused by disruption of your sleep, which are mostly the short and moderate term effects, and those caused by the apnea itself, which are largely the long term effects.

> There is, of course, a lot of overlap here. Chronic, long term disruption of sleep has additional effects beyond those we will discuss and signs of the long term effects can often be detected after a single night.

Sleepiness....

Most of the consequences of disrupted sleep are intuitively obvious. If you don't sleep well then you will be tired, sleepy and unrested the next day.

In fact, "excessive daytime sleepiness" or EDS, technically referred to as hypersomnolence, is traditionally recognized as the cardinal symptom of sleep apnea.

But not everyone gets sleepy and not everyone who is sleepy actually knows it!

> For example, it is not uncommon for someone to deny sleepiness during the day but on closer questioning to discover that she, or more typically he, drinks two or more **pots** of coffee during the day. And studies have shown that many nightshift workers fall asleep on the job without even realizing it.

> And many people do not distinguish between the feeling of sleepiness and the feeling of tiredness. Indeed, technically

there might be some overlap in the definition of these symptoms.

Besides the obvious inconvenience and unpleasantness of such sleepiness caused by sleep apnea, the first and major associated problem is safety.

In one study, drivers with an untreated diagnosis of sleep apnea were found to be twice as likely to have an auto accident over the next five years as the general population and **NINE TIMES** as likely as those whose sleep apnea was treated. One could infer from this study that there are many cases of undiagnosed sleep apnea in the general population, and this has been supported by epidemiological studies.

Memory and concentration difficulty....

Another consequence of disturbed sleep is memory and/or concentration difficulty. This is because sleep, actually a specific stage of sleep, is important in storing information in long term memory. And that stage of sleep is particularly disturbed by obstructive sleep apnea.

Longer term effects:

There are also consequences, usually longer term, caused by the sleep apnea independent of its effect on sleep. Before we go into these, we will digress a little to talk about what happens when you stop breathing in your sleep due to **obstructive** sleep apnea.

Remember, as stated above, obstructive sleep apnea occurs when you essentially suck your throat closed and obstruct your airway. But, think about it, nothing will make you panic quicker than having your air cut off. When that happens you will get an immediate response to fight for your breath. This is the "fight or flight" reflex, commonly referred to as a "surge of adrenalin", and scientifically referred to as "sympathetic activation" or "sympathetic nervous activation" or SNA. And, although it is a great response when you are caught in an alley with a mugger, or a bear is chasing you, it isn't a good response when you are trying to sleep because .....

The "fight or flight" response is just that. It prepares you to fight or run away by (among other things) increasing the force and rate of your heart's contractions, increasing your blood sugar, etc. For many people with moderate to severe sleep apnea, their heart is working harder when they are asleep than when they are awake.

And that is the way obstructive sleep apnea does much of its damage!

> People often focus on the reduced blood oxygen that occurs after they stop breathing. But, a normal, healthy, not overweight, middle-aged or younger adult, probably cannot hold his or her breath long enough for the blood oxygen drop significantly. In a clinical setting, these individuals may have severe apnea, with a high AHI, but have minimal desaturations. There is a reason for this but it's beyond the scope of this book. So.... The fight or flight response associated with sleep apnea may be independent of the oxygen level and is initially related to your brain determining that your airway is blocked.

> Don't get me wrong, the oxygen does matter. But, if the oxygen drops, it is just "icing on the cake" and another confounding factor making things even worse. In fact, research data tells us that the reduced oxygen levels also increase SNA and, furthermore, there is damage caused by repeated desaturations followed by returning to normal saturation, what is called the re-oxygenation injury.

> This is the reason you need CPAP for sleep apnea rather than just using supplemental oxygen. When people ask, I use the self-evident answer that the extra oxygen does no good if you don't breathe it in, but the more accurate answer is that obstructive sleep apnea damages your health even if your oxygen does not drop.

With this understanding of obstructive sleep apnea, what are some of the health consequences that we commonly see that can be traced to the apnea *per se*? These include:

Headaches, especially in the morning
High Blood Pressure or Hypertension
Congestive Heart Failure
Recurrence of Atrial Fibrillation/Flutter
Increased risk of heart attack or myocardial infarction
Increased risk of stroke
Poor control of blood glucose (sugar) in diabetics

All of these effects are due, wholly or in part, to the sympathetic
nervous activation (SNA), the "fight or flight" response, associated with
obstructive sleep apnea. Again, if you happen to have significant
blood oxygen desaturations associated with your apnea, all of these
problems are exacerbated but they can occur even without
desaturation.

Again, I do not want to ignore the desaturations but to
emphasize that the sympathetic activation occurs even without
the desaturation. The desaturation only makes the problem
worse.

Chapter 4

Who should be tested for sleep apnea and how is it diagnosed?

Sleep apnea is a very insidious disorder. Frequently the apnea sufferer has no idea that he or she has a sleeping problem. Instead, she or he attributes the symptoms to aging or weight or being "out of shape" or maybe to some other medical condition such as diabetes, depression, low thyroid levels, or medications.

The person with sleep apnea often considers himself a "champion" sleeper, saying that he can sleep all night then go right back to sleep after breakfast. For that reason, I believe there is a good reason to have a sleep study even if CPAP becomes an over-the-counter device.

Who....

Appendix II gives a questionnaire we have sometimes used during my talks to help people decide whether they should talk to their doctor about being evaluated for sleep apnea. There is also a statistically validated questionnaire, the "Berlin Questionnaire", that is generally recognized as a good indicator of the possibility of obstructive sleep apnea. The Berlin Questionnaire, however, requires "scoring" by the healthcare professional. There is another validated questionnaire often used by anesthesiologists called the STOP-BANG. The name comes from the questions about: **S**noring, **T**ired, **O**bserved apnea, high blood **P**ressure, **B**MI, **A**ge, **N**eck circumference, and **G**ender. In more general terms, you should be tested for sleep apnea if you:

Snore or have been told you stop breathing in your sleep

and, have one or more of the signs or symptoms below:

Tired or sleepy during the day or need lots of caffeine
Have high blood pressure

Have had a heart attack or stroke
Wake up multiple times during the night
Have trouble with concentration or memory
Have had a recent, unexplainable weight gain

Some people who have obstructive sleep apnea do not snore on a regular basis and some people just won't accept the word of family members that they snore. So if you don't snore, or don't admit it, but have one or more of the listed symptoms for no apparent reason, evaluation for sleep might be informative.

Of course, many people snore but do not have sleep apnea. Whether snoring always evolves into sleep apnea is debatable but there is little debate that it often does.

The only sure way to diagnose, or rule out, sleep apnea is with an in-the-lab sleep test. There are two basic types of sleep tests.

How: home studies....

In-home sleep tests (HST) are now approved for insurance coverage for CPAP. These have the advantage of being less expensive and the convenience of sleeping in your own home.

A major disadvantage is that most of these tests are unable to determine when you are awake versus when you are asleep. So breathing irregularities that are normal while awake, such as swallowing or speaking, might be misinterpreted as apnea resulting in an overestimation of the severity of apnea. Conversely, lying quietly in bed for a prolonged awake period might result in an underestimation of apnea severity.

For this reason, published guidelines recommend in-home studies only for people with a high probability of having sleep apnea. That is because the HSTs are good to confirm sleep apnea when obvious apnea exists but are not particularly good to "rule out" sleep apnea and confirm that it does not exist.

Home sleep tests have been around for a very long time, since the early nineties or so. When shown these devices my response was essentially the same as today: they will show what I really already know about the person after listening to his or her sleep and medical history and physical appearance. But it would not help with the person with primarily subtle hypopnea and those are the very people that CPAP may change the course of their lives for the better.

The guidelines further recommend HST only for those without significant medical comorbidities, such as heart problems, or comorbid sleep disorders. Unfortunately, it is arguably the presence of these comorbidities that constitutes a high probability of sleep apnea and these are the very people who want to be sure that a negative test really means they do not have sleep apnea. This is a point missed by many of the insurance companies which consider the HST as a "screening" test.

Disclaimer: We do provide HSTs from our sleep laboratory and the updated AASM Standards for Accreditation effective January, 2017, require all accredited sleep labs (now officially called a "facility") provide HSTs as well as all the laboratory based tests such as the multiple sleep latency test (MSLT) and the maintenance of wakefulness test (MWT).

Quality control standards for in home sleep studies call for them to be regularly compared to laboratory based studies. Many companies providing HST services to doctor's offices, however, may have no affiliation with a sleep laboratory for quality control purposes.

Another form of in-home "sleep test" that has been around for many years is simple oximetry. In the past it has been advocated by DME companies as a marketing tool. This is not considered a sleep study by accepted criteria and not accepted as an HST for the purposes qualifying for apnea treatment. It has all the disadvantages mentioned above for the in-home sleep studies with the added disadvantage of having no measure of breathing airflow. As explained earlier, sleep apnea *per se* is damaging to your health even without notable desaturations and oximetry would miss this entirely.

Increasingly, insurance companies are requiring HST for suspected sleep apnea, regardless of the shortcomings. This is largely driven by cost considerations in response to the suspected prevalence of undiagnosed sleep apnea.

A recent development is the use of "fitness monitors" to record sleep. These devices are based on movement measured by accelerometers and proprietary software. These devices are interesting novelties but are not sufficiently accurate for clinical use at this time. Studies vary but have shown that they are reasonably accurate for a good sleeper but inconsistently less accurate for poor sleepers. In the sleep field we are, of course, most often dealing with those with poor sleep.

How: lab based studies....

Sleep lab based sleep studies are considered the "gold standard" of sleep evaluations.

The studies are attended by a sleep technologist who monitors the testing and records observations throughout the entire night. The sleep lab accreditation standards specify the training and certification of the technologist and recommend one tech for every two test subjects under normal conditions. The presence of a technologist watching what is actually being recorded in real time is the cardinal advantage of the lab based tests and part of what makes it the standard.

Lab based studies record six channels of EEG data, along with eye movements and muscle tension, which allow the determination and staging of sleep. This assures the "sleep" in sleep apnea. It also helps your doctor know if the severity of your sleep apnea differs in various sleep stages.

Two channels of airflow using different technologies are recorded. Respiratory effort is recorded, both chest and abdomen, as is oximetry. With this data, respiratory events can be precisely defined and classified. Sleeping position is also monitored and the apnea/hypopnea index is determined by position.   The EKG and leg movements are also recorded.

In addition to more complete data and technologist observation, as described, an evaluation in a full sleep disorders center allows for the evaluation of comorbid sleep disorders, increasing the probability of a successful intervention.

There are two basic approaches used by sleep labs in diagnosing sleep apnea and initiating CPAP. These are referred to as "split-night" and "two-night" protocols and there is a legitimate debate among the proponents of each.

The split-night protocol calls for a baseline recording period, up to about two hours, to document sleep apnea, followed by a CPAP initiation period to determine the optimal CPAP pressure. The split-night has the advantage of only one night away from home and, consequently, lower cost. The disadvantage is that people often have trouble returning to sleep after starting the CPAP and even if they fall back asleep quickly, there is less time to determine the needed CPAP pressure than with a two-night approach.

The two-night protocol calls for an entire night of recording to document, and determine the severity of, the sleep apnea. This is followed by a full second night to initiate CPAP and determine the pressure setting. The disadvantage is, of course, increased time and expense. The two-night protocol has the advantage of determining the severity of sleep apnea across the entire night. Many people get worse as the night progresses, usually because they have more "REM" sleep in the early morning hours and their apnea is worse in REM sleep.

I once had a rather dramatic example of this. The gentleman had a high probability of sleep apnea so we planned a split-night study. After two hours of sleep, he had had no apnea or hypopnea so the technologist called me at home and we did not begin CPAP. By morning he had over six hundred events!

The two-night protocol, with the advantage of an entire night, will typically result in at least two more hours to optimize the CPAP pressure setting. There are published papers which show that a split-night is suitable for finding a single CPAP pressure setting for controlling the apnea. I prefer a two-night protocol because I find it better for finding a range of pressures for an auto-adjusting machine which, according to my data, results in better compliance.

Now let's turn our attention to some of the treatments for obstructive sleep apnea....

Chapter 5

Treatments for sleep apnea

By far, the most effective treatment for obstructive sleep apnea, and the only treatment that is consistently effective, is "positive airway pressure" or PAP, which is the topic of this book. This is because, as discussed in Chapter 2, obstructive sleep apnea is a multifactorial disorder. Again, the contributing factors to obstructive sleep apnea are:

> Overweight/Obesity
> Facial structure and anomalies
> Tissue elasticity
> Sleep stage and/or position
> Respiratory control and/or respiratory muscle factors
> Nasal congestion and/or allergies
> Cardiac status

All other treatments focus on a single contributing factor. If this single factor, such as the length of the palate or position of the jaw, is the only or even the major factor causing a particular case of sleep apnea, then treatment of this cause is likely to be effective. If on the other had there are, as commonly happens, multiple contributing causes for the apnea even in an individual, then treatment of any one of them uncovers another cause and is unlikely to be very effective.

Why PAP works so well....

PAP has the advantage of treating the **mechanism** of the sleep apnea rather than the **cause**. It is, therefore, consistently effective at controlling the apnea but does not cure the apnea.

> A good analogy is hypertension, high blood pressure, which is controlled but not cured by medication. If you stop taking your blood pressure medicine, the pressure will return to an elevated level. Treatment of sleep apnea with CPAP is like that.

Of course, it would be preferable to cure your sleep apnea and some people are able to do this, especially with surgery and/or weight loss and exercise. I will discuss the factors contributing to the success or failure of other sleep apnea treatments when these are covered in a later chapter.

The types of PAP....

Let's return to our discussion of PAP. There are several variations:

> Continuous Positive Airway Pressure or CPAP, referred to as "straight CPAP"
> CPAP with pressure relief, such as "Flex" or "EPR"
> Auto-adjusting CPAP or "AutoPAP" or "APAP"
> Defunct versions of CPAP such as "Demand" PAP or "DPAP"
> Bilevel PAP or BPAP ("BiPAP" is actually a brand name)
> Specialized forms: BiPAPautoSV, BiPAP AVAPS, VPAP Adapt SV, etc.

Throughout this book I will use PAP to refer generically to all the variations. However because CPAP, in all its versions, is by far the most common and many of the problems are common to all versions, often when I use the term CPAP the statement is equally applicable to the other forms of PAP, such as BiPAP or VPAP.

All versions of PAP deliver positive air pressure through a facial interface, commonly referred to as a "mask" even when it doesn't remotely resemble anything you would think of as a mask. People often confuse problems with their mask with problems with their machine.

It is necessary to determine where the problem is before it can be resolved.

There are probably forty or fifty different masks on the market, with more every year. There is a mask that will be comfortable for you. It might not be the first one you try, or the second one, or even the third or fourth one. We will discuss masks later.

Common alternative and adjunctive treatments....

Other common treatments for sleep apnea include:

Oral appliances, usually custom fit by your dentist

ENT and maxillofacial surgeries, such as:
> Uvulopalatopharyngeoplasty, known as UPPP or UP3
> Laser Assisted Uvulo-Pharyngeoplasty, or "LAUP"
> The "Pillar procedure", Somnoplasty, etc. These are proprietary procedures.
> Nose specific surgeries such as rhinoplasty, turbinectomy, etc.
> Less common procedures such as maxillomandibular or mandibular advancement, hyoid suspension, tongue reduction, tracheostomy, etc.
> Other Nasal treatment: Nose sprays or drops, Nasal expander strips

Weight loss through diet and exercise, medications, or bariatric surgery

> The recommendation of exercise is particularly interesting considering a published study which demonstrated that regular exercise, with both aerobic and "strength" components, for three months resulted in significantly improved sleep apnea even without significant weight loss. Although the subjects did not lose weight, they did lose body fat with a corresponding increase in muscle mass. The obvious inference from this study is that sustained regular exercise would result in further improvements in AHI. The unanswered question was whether the improvement came from the reduction or redistribution of body fat or from improved respiratory control.

Positional training to avoid sleeping on the back because many apnea suffers are worse on their backs.

Lifestyle changes: avoiding alcohol and/or sedating medications, quitting smoking, etc.

Less common because newer alternatives....

One new device applies a suction to the mouth to pull the palate down and the tongue forward and expand the posterior pharynx area.

Another approach is to position small pressure regulator valves over the nares producing a back pressure as you exhale. The device claims to have relatively little resistance to inhalation but more resistance to exhalation. The concept is that the back pressure keeps the airway open longer and may stabilize the respiratory control.

Another approach is a surgically implanted stimulator which triggers when it detects you begin to inhale and stimulates the muscles in your neck stabilizing the airway. The device can be turned on and off using a remote control. The procedure, although minor, is invasive with the associated risks.

Less common & outmoded alternatives....

Other, less common and/or outmoded treatments include: singing or voice exercises, playing some musical instruments, medication.

> The use of medication in treating obstructive sleep apnea is particularly interesting since the most commonly used medications were those that specifically reduced the amount of "REM" sleep you might have. The logic was that, since many people find that their apnea is worse in REM sleep, reducing the amount of REM would reduce the amount of apnea. Implicit in such an approach, however, is the assumption that REM sleep serves no useful purpose or that, at least, you need less than you normally get. As a "sleep expert" rather than a breathing expert, I believe the data shows that REM sleep is important.

This ebook and the video programs focus on adjusting to and tolerating PAP because it is the most common and, by far, the most effective treatment. We will cover many of the pros and cons of the common other treatments, and how to determine if they might be right for you, in a section near the end of the book. Several of them are also good adjuncts to your CPAP therapy.

Let's now return to the various versions of PAP and discuss them in more detail.

Chapter 6

Types of PAP machines

All versions of PAP work by maintaining a stable, open airway with a positive air pressure. In simplest terms, they consist of a blower or compressor, a delivery hose, and a "patient interface" or mask. They differ in how that pressure is managed both for effectiveness and for comfort.

Straight, old fashioned, CPAP....

First, there is straight CPAP: continuous positive airway pressure. This is the most basic of PAP treatments and is virtually unchanged in concept over the past quarter century. It delivers a constant level of positive air pressure throughout the breathing cycle.

> Technology has changed. The earlier commercial versions of CPAP utilized a constant pressure generator (blower) and controlled the pressure by use of a regulator valve. The valves were set at fixed pressures and had to be swapped out to change your pressure. This assured the CPAP user could not change the pressure.

> Newer machines use a microprocessor to maintain the pressure. Changing pressure is a simple panel entry or remotely by use of a modem.

Unfortunately, many people find it difficult to exhale against this pressure, particularly at higher pressure settings. There is probably no reason to maintain as high a pressure during exhalation as during inhalation. Fortunately, few doctors still order straight CPAP for their patients.

> Some insurance companies, especially with their "HMO" products, require that you use one of these primitive machines for a period, often three months, before allowing you to try a more sophisticated machine. This is probably the only residual

usage of straight CPAP but this is poor patient care and poor business. Studies have shown that the sooner the patient adapts to the CPAP, the more likely he or she is to use it long term and that consistent use of CPAP can reduce ancillary medical costs.

In days past these CPAP machines were noisy and the output air was uncomfortably warm. Today, even the simplest CPAP machines run quietly and coolly.

Bilevel PAP machines....

Next to come along were bilevel machines which vary the pressure according to the phase of the breathing cycle. "BiPAP" is a trademarked brand name for the original bilevel machine but is often used generically. Bilevel machines are also sometimes referred to as BPAP.

Although bilevel machines have some similarities to ventilators, and the more sophisticated versions are useful in treating some of the more complicated variants of sleep disordered breathing, they are not usually notably, if any, better than the modern CPAP machines for obstructive sleep apnea. Some people still find bilevel machines more comfortable than CPAP but most comfort issues are better managed using the expiratory relief versions discussed below.

Unfortunately, nothing works perfectly and people sometimes complain that the bilevel machine wants them to inhale while they are still trying to exhale. Or, conversely, they find that it does not detect when they are ready to inhale and fails to increase the pressure quickly enough.

This is probably the greatest shortcoming of bilevel machines in the treatment of obstructive sleep apnea.

Bilevel PAP machines are often beneficial for those with hypoventilation with, or without, obstructive sleep apnea. They are sometimes tried for central sleep apnea but this is usually not very effective, and even may be counterproductive, which should not be surprising considering the mechanism of central apnea. Use of a backup rate on a bilevel machine also does not usually help with central events, again because of the mechanism. (There are, however, specialized versions designed for central apnea discussed below.)

Expiratory relief....

The next level of sophistication, expiratory relief, came along around 2003 or 2004 to make exhalation easier.   Respironics developed the original version and called it "C-Flex" and was followed later by the ResMed version called "EPR" for expiratory pressure relief.

Both of these are trademarked names and they differ in the details of how the pressure changes over the breathing cycle. These pressure details are not really relevant to this discussion and will not be covered. In spite of the similarity to the proprietary name EPR, we will use the expression "expiratory relief" to refer to this feature generically.

Expiratory relief differs from bilevel PAP in a very important way.

The difference between bilevel and expiratory relief....

Bilevel machines reduce the pressure upon expiration and keep the pressure low throughout the expiratory phase. They then increase the pressure back to a higher level upon inspiration.

> The standard version waits until it detects that you are trying to breathe in before it increases the pressure. There is a timed version that increases the pressure to the inspiratory level after a defined time interval.

By contrast, CPAP machines with expiratory relief reduce the pressure at the beginning of the expiratory phase of the breathing cycle. They then gradually and smoothly return to the higher inspiratory pressure before the end of exhalation. Thus they provide full pressure support at the beginning of inspiration and avoid the problems sometimes associated with bilevel PAP machines.

Auto-adjusting PAP....

The next level of sophistication, auto-adjusting machines, has been in development for many years. These machines are supposed to automatically adjust the pressure level based upon the person's need. The current units from Respironics and ResMed also have expiratory relief.

Some doctors use the auto-adjusting feature to select a pressure which is then set for a fixed pressure, expiratory relief CPAP. There is a hybrid version which will auto-adjust for thirty days then revert to a fixed machine based on the results. The trial can be repeated as needed. Others use an auto-adjusting machine set for the maximum range of pressures and just let the machine "do its thing" as a permanent PAP therapy.

The other approach is to set the machine to a limited range of pressures determined by a lab based titration and utilize the auto-adjusting feature to accommodate the varying pressure requirement from night to night and during the night depending upon sleeping position, stage of sleep, and other factors. Such an approach can result in significant comfort improvements and make the PAP therapy more tolerable.

> To believe that these machines can reliably detect respiratory events with 100% accuracy, distinguish between obstructive and central events, and adjust the PAP level appropriately, is naive. But the newer auto-adjusting machines are much better at detecting and classifying respiratory events.

> If the testing in the sleep lab revealed a range of pressures, all of which appeared to adequately control the breathing, but which differed in sleeping position and sleep stages, then an auto-adjusting machine can be limited to work within that range as described above. This is the approach we have used for a number of years.

By design, of course, an auto-adjusting machine will result in less than perfect control of respiration because some respiratory events must occur for it to detect before it can raise the pressure. And the machines periodically lower the delivered pressure to determine if you still need that level. Thus, if an auto-adjusting machine controls the respiratory events completely it is because the very lowest pressure was sufficient.

> My philosophy has always been that a person using a machine 95% of the time that controls the 90% of the respiratory events when it is used is better than a machine that controls 100% of the events but is used 50% of the time.

PAP versions for special situations....

There are several specialized versions of PAP designed for specific, less common, more complicated types of sleep disordered breathing. These go by such names as:

> BiPAP S/T which includes a timed backup
> BiPAPautoSV for servoventilation BiPAP
> BiPAP AVAPS for Average Volume Assured Pressure Support
> VPAP ST which has a timed backup rate
> VPAP Adapt SV a servoventilation system

And, of course, others. We are not going to discuss these in detail, however, many of the tolerance problems we will discuss are applicable to these situations.

And an obsolete PAP version....

Finally, there are obsolete and defunct versions of PAP. The most notable, only because at least one insurance company (name withheld to protect the ignorant) is so out of touch that, as of the time of writing the first edition, they still referenced it in their coverage literature, is "demand positive airway pressure" or DPAP.

Other than communications from that insurance company, I last heard of this version sometime in the early 1990s. The concept was that it would quickly increase pressure to prevent respiratory events but, in practice, it simply awoke the patient. We will not discuss this version further.

A final thought on new PAP machines….

Early machines included a mechanical timer which recorded the cumulative number of hours of blower use. Modern machines include a recording protocol which keeps track of whether you are actually using the machine regularly. It still records how many hours the blower runs but it also records the number of hours you actually breathe on the machine on a night-to-night basis. The data may be recorded on a removable data card or may be transmitted by modem. This was driven by reimbursement requirements. In the US, most coverage (Medicare or private insurance) requires that you use your machine more than a specific minimum number of hours per night and a minimum number of nights per month.

> The most common minimum is 4 hours per night for 21 nights (70% of the nights) over 30 days within the first 90 days with the machine. These values are quite arbitrary and, although a reasonable initial goal, there is no objective, scientific supporting data that justifies their use as an inflexible constraint.

Most machines now also allow the user to review this data. It allows you to see how well your apnea is being controlled and whether you are reaching the required threshold for your machine to be paid for. Some machines also include an "app" for your phone or computer which lets you track your progress. The only caveat I would make about using the app or looking at your data is to not get discouraged if your progress seems too slow. Some people just take a while to get used to the machine. And do not get too worried about the insurance paying for your machine, there is a process for restarting the qualifying period although it may require another sleep test.

Chapter 7

Masks or patient interface

There are many different versions of masks...... versions that:

> cover the end of the nose
> cover the whole nose
> fit into the nostrils, sometimes called "nasal pillows" based on the first example
> cover the nose and mouth
> cover the mouth and also fit into the nostrils
> cover the whole face
> deliver the air into the mouth, like a scuba mask
> are held by the mouth and fit into the nose
> are made of cloth

People new to CPAP often confuse the mask with the machine itself. They will come into the sleep lab and say they want "the one that goes in the nose" while actually discussing the machine. They are also unaware that there are a number of masks from different manufacturers that fit that description.

Try several masks....

There is no reason a mask from one company cannot be paired with the CPAP machine from another company. Sometimes the medical equipment company will have a contract for a particular brand of CPAP machine and supplies, in which case they may not stock other makes of masks and will, therefore, have a bias.

This is especially true for the big national equipment companies. I think this is a mistake, both from a business perspective for the manufacturer and the supplier and for patient care. The equipment company should be able to provide you with whatever mask is comfortable enough for you to tolerate.

Some machines compensate for the known bias flow through the exhalation holes when reporting mask leak. This requires the machine to have data about that mask stored and, of course, the manufacturer only stores the data about their masks. This is another way they try to capture the mask business. This also makes the reported leak useful only as a relative value if you use another brand of mask and makes it difficult to compare leak numbers between machine brands.

As a practical matter, the pressure delivery through the various masks is consistent. That is not to say there are no differences but that the differences are usually minor enough to be addressed by your doctor's clinical judgment.

> People sometimes say they feel like they're getting more pressure through the nasal pillow type of mask, even though the machine setting is the same. In fact, the pressure is unchanged but the flow is increased.
>
> This happens because the nasal pillows deliver the pressure only into the nostrils, causing them to expand. Masks that cover the nose deliver the same pressure to the outside of the nose as well as into the nostrils and, therefore, don't cause this expansion of the nostrils.
>
> There is at least one (and I think only one) mask that delivers the pressure into the mouth like a scuba mask. Although the manufacturer claims that the pressure needed to control your apnea with this mask is the same as for a nasal mask, it is probable that this mask will differ somewhat in the required pressure. Nonetheless, empirical adjustment should be possible using the information downloaded from modern machines.

Your doctor may require that the medical equipment company get permission, or even a prescription, from him or her for any change in mask. This is done to be sure the doctor's clinical judgment is not circumvented. Sometimes the equipment company will have a policy that requires the doctor's order for any mask change. This is especially the case for the national companies if you want a mask brand they don't normally stock.

Other doctors will allow the equipment company to make any mask changes necessary as long as they communicate it to him or her for follow-up at your next appointment.

Although arguments can be made for either approach, from a practical point of view it is more time and cost efficient to let the equipment company select the mask that you will use.

People often ask which mask is best.

Masks are a very personal thing and there is no one "best" mask. The best mask is the one that fits comfortably with an acceptably small leak and that you will wear. A good analogy is shoes: the shoes that are best for you are not necessarily the same that are best for me. Other considerations include how easily the mask is disassembled and cleaned and how much trouble it is to put on and take off, especially during the night for a bathroom visit.

I do not endorse any specific mask. It is also impractical to discuss specific masks in a book, even an ebook, because of the variety and the constant introduction of new, and occasional retirement of old, models.

Chapter 8

Common problems associated with PAP usage

There are a number of common problems and challenges to adapting to and sleeping with CPAP. These include:

>Difficulty exhaling or unable to exhale
>The mask is uncomfortable, leaks, or causes sores on the face
>Unable to sleep all night with the CPAP
>Pulling the mask off during the night without knowing
>Opening the mouth or mouth breathing
>Difficulty falling asleep or staying asleep with the CPAP mask on
>Nasal congestion and/or a "runny nose"
>Ear or Sinus pain or discomfort
>Nasal obstruction; deviated septum

Other common problems include:

>Waking suddenly not breathing with the CPAP
>Central sleep apnea
>Chest pain or discomfort
>Claustrophobia
>Condensation in the hose, commonly called "rain out"
>Stomach bloating, belching/burping, or passing gas
>Air blowing in the eyes or out the ears
>Mask tickles or irritates the nose
>Air fills the cheeks then escapes through the mouth (the "chipmunk effect")
>Other sleep disorders, either coincidental or caused by the sleep apnea

If you have one or more of these problems, first be comforted that they are common problems and that many people have overcome them. I have often found that just knowing that a problem is common can help.

Reasons to not use PAP....

There **are** also some contraindications to using CPAP and some conditions in which CPAP should be used with caution. These contraindications must be addressed with straightforward guidelines and warnings before CPAP will be offered over the counter in the United States.

These contraindications include:

> Pneumothorax, a condition of air in the chest cavity but outside the lungs
> Heart failure that is acute and decompensated
> Epistaxis, a bloody nose, that is significant and massive, or a history of such
> Middle ear infection or perforated ear drum
> Respiratory distress syndrome or acute respiratory failure
> Sinusitis that is acute and severe

Your doctor should be aware of these and probably would not have prescribed CPAP without appropriate consideration of the risks and benefits. Some of the specialized versions of PAP have been developed especially for some of these conditions.

Chapter 9

Solutions to those problems

The solution to some of the problems are clear cut but some solutions are counter intuitive, exactly the opposite of what you might expect.

Difficulty exhaling or unable to exhale

This is a very common problem, especially at higher pressures. The first solution to this was bilevel PAP and, even today, some professionals consider bilevel to be the best solution. And for some people it is.

Around 2004, the expiratory relief option was added to CPAP. As mentioned above, expiratory relief differs from bilevel in that the pressure returns more gradually to the inspiratory level and without waiting for the user to begin inhaling. I have generally found the expiratory relief to be a better choice for this particular problem if the person has straightforward obstructive sleep apnea.

Auto-adjusting PAP may also be easier to exhale against because the pressure may be lower for much of the night.

Mask is uncomfortable, leaks, or causes sores on the face

As discussed above, there are many, many options for masks and the one you will find comfortable may not be the one someone else finds comfortable. The most obvious cause of an uncomfortable mask is the "wrong" mask for your face.

This is a common problem with some of the low priced insurance policies that mandate your CPAP machine and mask be shipped to you and with a medical equipment company that would provide such poor service. Medicare, unfortunately, has been considering going to this approach for a number of years and, as I write this, the concept continues to be on the table. This is a short-sighted approach and, although it might work for an insurance company that can eventually dump you onto another company, it makes no sense for Medicare which has someone basically for the rest of his/her life.

The bottom line is that you should have the benefit of a face-to-face meeting with an experienced sleep tech or respiratory therapist to properly fit the mask and instruct you on the operation and care of your machine. The mask manufacturers provide sizing gauges to help select the proper size but it can only be used by a face-to-face meeting.

> This is where I show my bias: why would an insurance company, or Medicare, want to pay for a piece of equipment but provide it with such poor support that a significant percentage of users will find it intolerable? The easiest way to cut cost is to reduce service and when medical equipment companies have to compete on cost alone, service is the first thing to suffer.

The tech or therapist should fit the mask to you in as nearly a normal sleeping situation as possible. You should be lying down, not sitting up. If you wear dentures and take them out at night, the mask should be fit with your dentures removed. If you sleep with rollers in your hair, the mask should be fit with rollers in your hair.

The next most common reason for mask discomfort is adjusting the headgear too tightly, usually to prevent leaks. The mask should not be so tight that it causes sores, or tenderness, on the face. Usually the mask is strapped on overly tight in an attempt to stop a leak. Often this is done by the user even with a mask that was properly fit by the therapist. Sometimes it is done to compensate for a poor mask choice or fit. The bottom line is: if it has to be uncomfortably tight to control the leak, it's the wrong mask for your face.

> What is important to realize is that most modern CPAP machines can compensate for a minor leak. In fact, the leak is likely to disturb the user long before the CPAP machine cannot handle it. Interestingly, the most sophisticated CPAP machines, the auto-adjusting machines, are somewhat less tolerant of leak because it can deceive their event detection

program. This may limit the utility of an auto-adjusting CPAP for some people.

Unable to sleep all night with the CPAP

This problem is so common that we probably shouldn't even list it as a problem but as a normal stage in adapting to CPAP. If after two to four weeks of sleeping with the CPAP mask and machine, you find that you make it only about three or four hours before you just have to pull it off, don't give up, you may be on your way to CPAP satisfaction.

> Yes, some people have absolutely no problem adapting to CPAP. They wake up after their night in the lab asking how soon they will get their machine, and sleep through the night with it from the very first night. Although this is not uncommon, it is certainly not the norm.

There is a normal, physiologic reason for waking after a few hours unable to return to sleep with the CPAP.

> Under normal circumstances, most people will get their deepest sleep in the first three hours or so (the first couple "sleep cycles"). During this time it is often easy to tolerate a new sleeping condition, such as a mask on the face, simply because the drive to sleep is so strong and the sleep is so deep. After this period of deep sleep, it can be challenging to stay asleep with any new condition.

You should determine if there is a specific reason for you waking up such as nasal congestion, water in the hose or mask, a leaking mask, or even noisy neighbors. I can't make any recommendations on how to handle the neighbors, but I will address the other, CPAP related, problems.

Warning:

> If you have uncontrolled high blood pressure, have severe heart disease such as congestive heart failure, a malignant arrhythmia, multiple heart attacks, or are at high risk for stroke, it is very important that you adapt to your PAP as quickly as

possible so you can sleep through the night with it.

Do not take this section to mean that you do not need to work toward sleeping all night on your machine, rather, understand that many people struggle at first. Talk to your doctor about the problems you are having sleeping with the PAP. He or she may offer you a sleeping pill for a couple weeks to help you adapt but remember, long-term use of most sleeping pills in not recommended.

Pulling the mask off during the night

There are two main reasons you might pull your mask off while asleep during the night. Here I am referring to pulling the mask off without knowing it so that you find it laying on the floor in the morning with no memory of pulling it off. The two common reasons are:

> Mask discomfort
> Nasal congestion

We have discussed mask discomfort in other sections and all the remedies apply here as well. Generally, if the mask becomes uncomfortable during the night without being notably uncomfortable at the beginning of the night, the most likely causes are:

> a poorly fitting mask
> a mask that is adjusted too tightly
> the mask has shifted on your face

We've already discussed the issues of mask fit and tightness. Shifting on the face may be caused by a poorly fitting mask but may also be caused by your pillow.

> There are pillows available that have been specifically designed with contours to avoid shifting the CPAP mask. Talk to your medical equipment company about this, they may carry them in stock although it is unlikely that your insurance company will pay for it.

Nasal congestion is less obvious as a cause of pulling the mask off, but it is very common, especially if you are opening your mouth during the night.

> Think about it. You can't get enough air through your nose because it is congested. You don't know you're congested, because you are asleep, but you do feel something on your face. Your instinctive response will be to pull it off.

The first thing to do for nasal congestion during the night is to increase the humidifier setting, either turning the temperature up or selecting a higher humidity range depending upon the model.

> Probably the most common reason for nasal congestion on CPAP, assuming you didn't have a nasal congestion problem without CPAP, is mechanical irritation of the nasal tissue from the cool, dry air. Your doctor may refer to this as "vasomotor rhinitis".

Often the nasal congestion begins after you open your mouth during your sleep. Sometimes adjusting the humidifier as suggested will solve this problem but you may need a chin strap to help you keep your mouth closed. Fortunately, as you learn to sleep with the CPAP pressure, you may not need the chin strap on a permanent basis. Another option is to use a "full face" mask that covers both the nose and mouth but, then, you are unlikely to learn to keep your mouth closed.

If adjusting the humidifier, and maybe using a chin strap or full face mask, does not solve the problem of pulling the mask off, and it does seem to be related to nasal congestion, talk to your doctor about the appropriateness of using a nasal steroid spray.

> Nasal steroid is now available over-the-counter (OTC) and there are still prescription nasal steroids. **Do not** try a prescription steroid spray not prescribed to you. If your doctor does suggest a nasal steroid, whether OTC or prescription, use it as recommended. Do not use it more frequently or longer without your doctor's instruction to do so.

Of course, if you have a deviated nasal septum, it will take even less congestion to give you a problem and the doctor may suggest surgical correction. In my experience, correction of a deviated septum is the most consistently helpful of surgical procedures.

Opening the mouth or mouth breathing

One of the most common, and challenging, problems associated with CPAP usage is mouthbreathing. Breathing through the mouth is very common in untreated obstructive sleep apnea.

> As the airway obstructs and the airflow diminishes, the apnea sufferer instinctively opens his or her mouth to get more air. Although the obstruction is in the pharynx, not at the mouth, opening the mouth helps by reducing the resistance he or she must pull against. With less resistance, less forceful inhalation is necessary reducing the tendency for the airway to collapse.

This habitual pattern often continues when starting CPAP, and is particularly annoying because the air rushes out the mouth, sometimes with enough noise to disturb the bedpartner. Most CPAP machines can adapt to the increased flow of air in through the nose and out the mouth, which to the machine is a leak, and maintain the prescribed pressure. Ironically, the most sophisticated CPAP machines, the auto-adjusting machines, are more susceptible to leak, including mouthbreathing, than the simpler models because they use airflow changes to detect respiratory events.

For many people, as their sleeping brain learns that they actually get more air by keeping the mouth closed, they stop breathing through the mouth. So, give it some time, maybe with the help of a chin strap, and see if the mouthbreathing stops on its own.

In the meantime, experiment with the humidifier setting, generally increasing the setting for more humidity or heat. As discussed above, sometimes nasal congestion begins with mouthbreathing, but as the nasal congestion progresses and it becomes harder to pull air through the nose, the mouth opens even more.

> One of the physiologic functions of the nose is to warm and humidify the air on its way to the lungs. By the time the air

reaches the lungs, it must be warmed to approximately 98.6° and humidified to 100%. When the mouth opens and an abnormally high volume of air flows through the nose, the nose simply cannot keep up and responds with congestion.

A common misconception is that a humidifier is unnecessary in areas, such as where I live on the Gulf Coast, where nighttime humidity is in the upper 90's and temperatures in the mid 80's during the summer. But almost everyone has air conditioning now and so the actual ambient indoor conditions, the conditions you are sleeping in, are typically temperatures in the 60's or 70's with a humidity of about 50%.

Similar to nasal congestion, nasal obstruction caused by a deviated septum or other anatomical abnormality can result in mouth breathing. If you suspect this is your problem, discuss it with your doctor and consider seeing an ENT specialist.

> In this case, the resistance to airflow is constant but is simply too great to force the air through and the mouthbreathing was probably noticed before starting CPAP. A surgical approach is usually necessary.

As discussed above, a chin strap may be necessary to help keep the mouth closed and should be the next option tried. The chin strap may only be needed for a few months as you subconsciously learn, in your sleep, that you get more air without opening your mouth.

Sometimes, as a last resort, changing the pressure may help. It is not always obvious whether the pressure should be increased or decreased so it's essential that it be done only upon your doctor's order. Raising the pressure may force sufficient air through the nose to eliminate the drive to open the mouth. Or it may result in increased mechanical irritation and nasal congestion, increasing the tendency to open the mouth even more. On the other hand, reducing the pressure may reduce the irritation and congestion and, therefore, the drive to open the mouth. Keep in mind, however, that your doctor selected that pressure for a reason and may not consider it advisable to change.

Difficulty falling asleep or staying asleep with the CPAP

This is a very common problem with three basic causes.

> Unfamiliarity with the experience
> Mask discomfort
> Too much or too little pressure

We have all experienced difficulty falling or staying asleep after making a change in our sleep environment. This can be as minor as not using a fan in the fall after using it all summer or rearranging the furniture. It can be as major as moving halfway around the world.

Sleeping with a mask on your face may be one of the most dramatic changes in sleep environment you will ever experience. And this can manifest itself as insomnia.

> One "trick" in learning to sleep with CPAP is to prepare your machine and fit the mask to your face at bedtime but not actually put it on until after you first doze off. This, of course, is dependent upon you waking briefly but many people drift in and out of sleep before finally remaining asleep for an extended period. After you become used to sleeping with the CPAP, you should be able to fall asleep easily with it on.

Like the insomnia associated with other changes in the sleep environment, time will often solve the problem as you become used to the new conditions. Your doctor may prescribe a sleeping pill for up to a couple weeks to help with this but remember, it is very easy to become dependent upon the sleeping pill.

> By the way, your sleep doctor may refer to your insomnia as DIMS for "difficulty initiating and maintaining sleep" or by just the component of insomnia you have. This may be abbreviated as DIS or DMS. Other expressions are "sleep initiation insomnia" or "sleep maintenance insomnia".

Mask discomfort is a major challenge to falling asleep and staying asleep, but mask discomfort should be addressed even if it doesn't cause insomnia. Talk to your doctor and the therapist at your medical equipment company about this.

The mask manufacturers often give the medical equipment companies replacements for any mask you reject within thirty days so don't be shy about asking for a replacement. The bottom line is, you should not be expected to sleep with an uncomfortable mask.

> Some equipment companies act like they are doing you a favor by exchanging masks in the first thirty days. Some, especially online companies, even charge you for the "insurance" that you can exchange your mask. This is ironic since they may get a full refund on the rejected mask!

Either too much or too little pressure can make it difficult to sleep. Especially in the case of sleep initiation, the sleep techs and respiratory therapists have a tendency to place the blame on too much pressure, however, it can be just as hard to fall asleep with too little pressure.

Generally, too much pressure will lead to insomnia due to difficulty exhaling. As discussed above, the first thing to try is more expiratory relief. Too little pressure will lead to insomnia due to feelings of "air hunger" or struggling to breathe in.

Talk to your doctor and the therapist from the equipment company about any insomnia problems you feel might be caused by pressure but try to think about whether it is too much or too little pressure. The therapist may discuss this with your doctor but will need the doctor's order to make any change.

Nasal congestion and/or a "runny nose"

One of the most common problems people face in learning to sleep with CPAP is nasal congestion and/or rhinorhea commonly called a "runny nose". You may experience both, with congestion during the night and a runny nose in the morning. Often the CPAP user will complain that the machine gave him or her a "cold" or a "sinus infection" and sometimes this is even after the very first night.

We've already discussed nasal congestion associated with simple mechanical irritation but, for completeness, will have a brief review in this section.

As discussed above, your nasal congestion may be due to vasomotor rhinitis. This is caused by the mechanical irritation of the nasal mucosa by the relatively cool dry air delivered from the CPAP machine. Of course, the air from the CPAP is neither cooler nor drier than the room air. But it is delivered under pressure and can, therefore, result in a significantly greater flow volume. This is particularly a problem if you open your mouth so the increased airflow moves through your nose and out your mouth.

If this is the source of your congestion and/or rhinorhea, try the suggestions made above in the sections on opening your mouth and on pulling the mask off. Specifically, try increasing the humidifier setting (either heat or humidity level depending upon the model) and adding a chin strap or full face mask if necessary.

There are other sources of nasal congestion and rhinorhea.

First, there is a daily or circadian rhythm to nasal symptoms. Normally, there is a nocturnal or nighttime increase in inflammatory cells in the nasal mucosa. This leads to a naturally occurring, nightly increase in nasal congestion and rhinorrhea in the morning.

You may have been aware of this even before starting CPAP. Many people notice it as nasal congestion and/or a runny nose in the morning for awhile after getting up.

What can you do about it?

The first thing to try is to flush the nasal mucosa with saline (salt water) before going to bed. Sterile saline nasal spray is available at the drug store as an over-the-counter product. Spray into your nose and then blow your nose thoroughly, possibly repeating several times.

If this doesn't help, you may need a nasal steroid spray. You should to talk to your doctor about this, but a nasal steroid is now available over-the-counter. There are also prescription nasal steroids which allow insurance coverage. Steroids may not be appropriate for all people, so whatever you do, don't use someone else's prescription and if you use an over-the-counter product, be sure to read the enclosed instructions and warnings. Follow the instructions.

Ear or Sinus pain or discomfort

Air trapping in the sinuses or middle ear can result in pressure and/or pain. And the pain can be intense. This is generally due to inadequate pressure equalization caused by congestion and can usually be managed.

You should discuss this problem with your doctor. Usually, your doctor will first try medication such as a nasal steroid spray. All the cautions about using nasal sprays discussed above pertain to this situation also. Depending upon your exact circumstances surgery may be indicated.

It may be possible to lower your CPAP pressure, or use expiratory relief to attain a lower average pressure. This may result in less air trapping and discomfort or pain. But remember, your doctor selected the pressure for a reason and it may not be possible to lower your prescription. Do not try to change your pressure yourself.

Nasal obstruction; deviated septum

Nasal obstruction refers to restricted airflow through the nose due to anatomical factors such as a deviated septum. It is constant, day and night. And it can absolutely limit, or totally prevent, your ability to tolerate CPAP.

By contrast, nasal congestion occurs from swelling of the nasal mucosa and varies throughout the day and night and from time to time. Many things can contribute to this including allergies and mechanical irritation. As discussed, nasal congestion may respond to reducing the contributing factors or to nasal steroids. Of course, you may have both a nasal obstruction and nasal congestion and their effects will be additive.

Generally, nasal obstructions are amenable to surgical correction. Correction of a nasal obstruction is, arguably, the most effective surgery commonly performed in the treatment of obstructive sleep apnea.

> Again, the nose has the narrowest cross sectional area of the entire respiratory system and thus is a point of high resistance. Any increase of cross sectional area at this point may thus result in a greater reduction of resistance than elsewhere.

Whether a nasal obstruction is your problem and whether there is a reasonable surgical option is something only your doctor can answer. Be sure to discuss the probability of success, and what is considered a success, as well as the risks and length of the recovery period with your doctor.

Waking suddenly not breathing on CPAP

A common problem encountered in the early stages of CPAP usage is the experience of waking suddenly, aware that you are not breathing. This is usually probably associated with a central apnea, a cessation of breathing effort. Sometimes the emergence of central apnea during your initial CPAP trial in the sleep lab limits the pressures that can be used. If there are enough events your apnea may be reclassified as "complex" sleep apnea.

> There is some question concerning the cause of these central respiratory events. It may be an example of, or similar to, the Hering-Breuer reflex which limits the extent of inspiration. The reflex is triggered by the stretch receptors in the chest which essentially tell the brain that the chest has expanded as far it should. Or it may be due to a gradual shift in the bicarbonate level in the blood to compensate for the nightly increase in carbon dioxide, which alters the respiratory control.

> It is quite possible that the isolated events that commonly wake people when beginning CPAP are caused by the former, and

the frequent events resulting in complex apnea is caused by the latter. That the central apnea worsens as the pressure often increases complex apnea confuses things but, either way, both the isolated events and the complex apnea will usually diminish with continued use of CPAP.

You may not have experienced central events while in the sleep lab, or they may have been rare and you were unaware of them. Once you have your CPAP home, however, these may occasionally become so long in duration as to awaken you suddenly from an otherwise sound sleep. Fortunately, this problem will normally resolve itself in time but it can certainly be troubling when it occurs.

Some medications or illicit drugs can lead to central apnea, either by reducing respiratory drive or by suppressing the arousal response. This should be discussed with your doctor.

Chest pain or discomfort

Chest pain or discomfort caused by using CPAP is usually chest wall pain related to the expansion of the chest by the pressure. In simplest terms, you haven't been breathing in as deeply in a long time and the mechanical stretch of the chest wall results in discomfort or even pain. This may occur along with the stretch induced isolated central events described above and, similarly, should resolve itself within a couple weeks. However ....

Warning: Chest pain or discomfort can also be related to more serious conditions involving your heart and/or lungs. If you have chest pain when you use your CPAP, especially if it is severe, talk to your doctor about it immediately.

Claustrophobia

One of the concerns most commonly expressed when first faced with the prospect of CPAP is claustrophobia. Often this is founded on a fear of suffocation when something is on the face. Certainly, a fear of being unable to get enough air is reasonable for a person suffering from obstructive sleep apnea. Fortunately, there are some things you can do to help alleviate the claustrophobia associated with CPAP usage, and most the time we have been able to overcome the problem. If you are worried about claustrophobia, try these suggestions:

1. The first thing to do, before you even try a CPAP, is to remind yourself that it will be supplying air. So suffocation is not really a concern. Remind yourself of this over and over, multiple times per day. Try to change your mindset.

2. Work with the sleep lab, prior to your CPAP trial, to find the best mask for you. You want to determine which factors contribute the most to your claustrophobia and try to avoid or minimize these.

There are a number of considerations:

> Does the size of the mask on your face contribute to your claustrophobic feelings? Or, does the headgear holding the mask contribute more to your feelings of claustrophobia? Is the tightness on your face the problem? Is it the feeling of the mask? Or is it the sight of the mask when you open your eyes?

> There a many mask designs and each of these problems have been addressed by at least one of them. Remember, there are masks that cover all of your nose, masks that cover just the end of your nose, masks that cover your nose and mouth, and masks that cover your whole face. There are masks that go in your nostrils, and masks that cover your mouth and go in your nostrils.

> There is a mask that blows in your mouth. There are masks with complicated headgear, masks with minimal headgear, and a mask with almost no headgear that you hold with your mouth. There is a cloth mask. There are masks that seal to the face with minimal tightness.

> If the mask itself is the source of your claustrophobia, there is probably a mask that will be tolerable because someone else has had the same problem before and the mask designers have

addressed it. Sometimes it is not the mask you would first think.

3. Next, you want to work on acclimation to the mask.

Hold your mask in your hand, without the headgear, and bring it up to your face, holding it in position for a few seconds to a minute or so. Do not hold it so long that you start to panic. This can be done while you are distracted with something else such as watching television and should be done several times per day. The more often you do this the faster you will adapt. And you might never adapt if you only do it once a day.

Do this first without the machine and hose connected to the mask. Be sure the hose is not attached or you will be rebreathing your exhaled carbon dioxide.

Once you are comfortable holding just the mask to your face, repeat the process with the CPAP machine connected and turned on so that it is supplying air. Set the expiratory relief at the maximum. Be sure the machine is on or you will be rebreathing carbon dioxide.

You want to continue doing this until you reach the point that you are comfortable holding the mask on your face indefinitely with the machine providing pressure. It may take you several days or even a week or two to reach this point, but keep trying.

Next, you want to actually put the mask on with the headgear. Again, do this while awake and do not leave it on until you start to panic. Again, start without the hose attached to the mask and then with the hose and the machine turned on. Do it multiple times a day until you are able to wear it, indefinitely, while distracted.

Only at this point are you ready to start trying to sleep with the mask. (A video shows the process at www.practicalhealthstrategies.com "online programs".)

4. Your doctor may offer you a tranquilizing or sedating medication to

help you during the adaptation phase. This is a perfectly reasonable approach. But remember, these medications usually make your respiratory events last longer so your ultimate goal should be to adapt to the CPAP machine and mask and discontinue the medication.

Condensation in the hose

Condensation of water in the hose, often referred to as "rain out", is a common problem with humidified CPAPs. The heated water chamber, combined with the extra surface area of a corrugated hose, makes a great "still".

You might be able to turn the heat down on your humidifier. On some newer units the temperature is not directly set by the user, instead the setting is for a humidity range rather than a temperature or heat setting and the machine compensates for the room temperature to assure the set humidity range. These units have less of a problem with condensation but it still occurs.

But, you selected that humidifier setting based on comfort and comfort is the ultimate goal. There are three things you can do to reduce the problems associated with condensation:

> 1. Place your CPAP unit on the floor next to the bed, without any low points in the hose, so that any condensation tends to run back down the hose into the humidifier chamber.

> 2. Insulate the hose with a cloth sleeve. These may be available from your medical equipment company or you may have to make one yourself. Regardless, your insurance company is unlikely to pay for this.

> If your mask orients the hose such that it runs down from your face, the hose can be placed under your bedcovers to accomplish the same thing. This is particularly successful if the CPAP machine is on the floor, as suggested above.

> 3. Try a heated hose. Most modern CPAP machines have a heated hose option from the manufacturer. There is also an aftermarket heated hose that can be used on any brand of

CPAP. This is an effective, but more expensive, solution that may not be covered by your insurance.

Stomach bloating, belching/burping

Bloating and belching is a common, and challenging, problem with CPAP. There are no sure fixes for this but things you can try include:

1. Reduce the average pressure: If you have an expiratory relief machine, increasing the relief to the maximum will reduce the average pressure and may reduce the bloating. Similarly, this may be less of a problem with a bilevel machine and bloating may be considered a "CPAP failure" to qualify for a bilevel machine for insurance purposes.

Your doctor may approve a lower CPAP setting for you but, remember, he or she picked the pressure for a reason and a lower pressure may not be effective for you. Talk to your doctor about the problem.

2. Sleep on your side. You may find that you have less bloating on your side than on your back and it may be different on one side than the other. Experiment with sleeping position.

3. Raise your head, either by blocks under the bed or on multiple pillows. This may result in less air trapping by the stomach. It may also reduce your pressure requirement resulting in lower pressures if you are on an auto-adjusting machine.

Air blowing in the eyes or out the ears

Air blowing in the eyes is usually a mask fit problem. You may need a different mask design, a different mask size, or just an adjustment of your mask. Talk to the therapist or sleep tech at the medical equipment company.

The therapist should fit the mask to you while you are in your normal sleep position (eg. lying down, on your back, side, and/or stomach) and sleep condition (eg. dentures in or out, hair rollers, face creams, etc.).

Another way that you might experience air blowing into your eyes is through the nasolacrimal tear ducts which normally drain tears from the eyes into the nose. Talk to your doctor about it if you think this is the source of your problem. Lowering the pressure may reduce, or eliminate, this problem but, again, the pressure was selected for a reason and a lower pressure may not be effective for you. There is a mask, the "total face" mask, that covers the whole face, including the eyes, which should solve the problem.

> On first looking at a total face mask you might think that air blowing in the eyes would be more of a problem with this mask. But with the entire face under the mask there is no net pressure gradient to cause the air to move toward, over, or into the eyes and no pressure gradient from one end of the tear duct to the other.

Air blowing out your ears may mean you have a perforated eardrum or "tubes" in the ears. Talk to your doctor and an ENT evaluation may be needed.

The mask tickles or irritates your nose

Mask irritation can be as simple as mechanical irritation or it can be the result of either contact or allergic dermatitis.

Mechanical irritation may require a change in mask type or fit. A common example of this problem is irritation of the inner surface of the nose by a pillow type mask. This problem is also common with poor mask fit or adjustment.

A dermatitis may respond to an over-the-counter hydrocortisone cream applied to the face at the site of the dermatitis or to the mask itself. The cream may, however, cause chemical deterioration of the mask seal. Be sure to follow the instructions on the package and tell your doctor about it on your next visit.

Some people have found relief using a lubricating and moisturizing jelly such as Vaseline® or K-Y®, however, these may also be incompatible with some mask materials.

Air fills the cheeks then escapes through the mouth

This is a common problem, sometimes referred to as the "chipmunk" problem. Some people find it amusing but some find it quite annoying because it often wakes them up. The basic cause of the problem is air entering the mouth from the pharynx because of an inadequate seal.

Keeping the mouth moist may help but may not completely control the problem. This works by creating a gasket like effect around the tongue and palate. Try a higher humidifier setting. Also, placing the tongue firmly against the roof of the mouth and the back surface of the front teeth may help.

Other sleep disorders

If you have another sleep disorder, either coincidental or developed secondary to your sleep apnea, it can be a challenge to getting used to sleeping with CPAP. It can also limit the benefit that you perceive from your CPAP. Since the last edition of this ebook, the classification of sleep disorders has revised the insomnia classifications. What was once independent disorders are better described as subtypes of the disorders chronic or short-term insomnia. The subtypes are relevant for our discussion.

Some of the more common sleep disorders and subtypes that you may have in addition to your sleep apnea, and which may limit your ability to tolerate CPAP or the benefit you experience from it are:

1. **Inadequate sleep hygiene**: This is a subtype of insomnia and refers to the sum total of behaviors that negatively impact your quality of sleep. Often, this may be a result of inappropriate responses to the poor sleep quality caused by the sleep apnea. Some of the counterproductive behaviors commonly adopted by sleep apnea suffers include:

Dozing in the evening before bedtime
Excessive caffeine consumption
Random napping during the day
Excessive time in bed attempting to get "enough sleep"
Evening alcohol consumption attempting to improve sleep
onset, but which actually increases the sleep fragmentation and
worsens the sleep apnea

2. **Shift Work Disorder**: This is included in the Circadian Rhythm
Sleep-Wake Disorders and can present as insomnia or as sleepiness.
Shiftworkers, because of the disruption of their "biological clock", often
experience light and fragmented sleep and/or sleepiness or fatigue
during their waking hours. CPAP can further increase the sleep
fragmentation for shiftworkers increasing the time it takes to develop
adequate sleep quality on the machine.

Furthermore, sleepiness and/or fatigue are common symptoms of
sleep apnea. Any residual sleepiness or fatigue that is due to the
shiftwork, rather than the apnea, will limit the perception of
improvement often described by new CPAP users.

3. **Hypnotic (sleeping or anxiety pill) dependency**: Many sleep
apnea sufferers have developed a dependence on sleeping
medications prior to being diagnosed with sleep apnea. This often
occurs when the person describes poor sleep to his or her doctor in
terms that, to the doctor, sound more like insomnia. Use of sleeping
or anxiety medication may fall within the insomnia category or as a
central hypersomnia.

Sleeping medications will worsen sleep apnea especially by
prolonging the respiratory events. This can usually be controlled by
the CPAP but may affect the required pressure. Sleeping medications
also frequently result in nonrestorative sleep, resulting in sleepiness or
fatigue the next day and limiting the benefit that a new CPAP user
might perceive. Fortunately, many doctors today will no longer
prescribe sleeping medications without first having a sleep lab
evaluation.

4. **Psychophysiological insomnia**: "Psychophysiological" refers to a

specific subtype of insomnia in which psychological arousal leads to physiological arousal which results in insomnia.

It is commonly associated with stress, but is particularly challenging when the insomnia itself becomes the stressor which leads to the psychological arousal. This type of insomnia usually manifests itself as a sleep onset insomnia and can severely limit the ability to fall asleep on CPAP especially when first starting out. It may also contribute to a sleep maintenance insomnia.

Your sleep doctor should be familiar with all of these sleep disorders and subtypes, as well as the over sixty other sleep disorders, and will have recommendations depending your specific circumstances. It is important that you discuss all your sleep problems with your sleep specialist in order to maximize tolerance of and benefit from CPAP.

Chapter 10

Frequently Asked Questions

Do I have to use my CPAP all the time, even when I nap?

The simple answer is: "Yes, you should." Remember that the damage caused by obstructive sleep apnea occurs because of the repeated sympathetic nervous system activation and this will occur on even a short nap.

What if I have a cold?

Unfortunately, if you are congested with a cold you may not be able to tolerate your CPAP until you are better. To make matters worse, the congestion from a cold will likely increase the severity of your sleep apnea.

Changing to a full-face mask that covers both the nose and mouth may help. A nasal decongestant spray may help, and this is an appropriate use for a decongestant, but check with your doctor beforehand. These sprays are contraindicated for people with high blood pressure and that includes many people with sleep apnea. Decongestant nose sprays can, also, be quite addictive to your nose.

Is it noisy?

Years ago, CPAP machines were noisy, CPAP masks were noisy and, to make matters worse, the air was hot. Today's machines are very quiet and they've learned how to vent the air quietly from the mask. The machines no longer run hot, either

So any noise is usually just airflow from the mask associated with the changes as you breathe in and out, and that is usually minimal. Of course, if you choose an older design of mask for

reasons of comfort, it may produce more noise as the air vents
out.

What about travel, can I take it on an airplane?

Modern CPAP machines are small, light, and come with a
convenient carrying case, usually with a shoulder strap. Most
people carry their CPAP machine with them as a "carry on"
when flying and, yes, the US TSA is familiar with CPAP. They
will probably ask you to open the case and let them inspect it.

Just in case, it might be helpful to have some paperwork
showing that the machine is actually yours. This could be the
billing paperwork you get from the medical equipment company
or a copy of your sleep study recommending a CPAP. I've
never actually heard of anyone needing this.

If you are traveling to a place at a higher or lower altitude than
where you usually use your CPAP machine, it may have to be
adjusted in order to deliver the proper pressure. Some new
machines can do this automatically but some require you to
make the change. This information should be in the manual
supplied with your machine but check this out with your medical
equipment company to be sure.

Do I need an adapter to use it in Europe?

Most modern CPAP machines are able to automatically analyze
the power source, both voltage and frequency, and adjust. Be
sure to verify for your specific machine. You may need an
adapter for the plug itself.

Can I take it camping with me?

That depends on what you call camping. If you're going
backpacking in the Andes, probably not. But if you are doing
the typical camper trailer, sure. You need to be sure that if you
use a generator or inverter that the waveform is acceptable.
There are line conditioners that will assure this for you.

There are compact battery powered CPAPs available. The battery charge is usually only good for one night so you will need a way to recharge it. There are also batteries available for common home CPAP machines but, again, keeping them charged may be a challenge.

How often should I get a new mask?

Your CPAP mask will deteriorate with time and your insurance will probably buy you a new one on a regular basis. This may be as often as once every three months or as rarely as once a year. If you have really bad insurance, it may not cover replacement supplies.

Even if your mask has not worn out at the time the medical equipment company says you qualify for a replacement, I suggest you get at least one as a backup. It can be very unpleasant if your mask breaks right at bedtime one night. You might also want to have a backup mask of a different design from your regular mask in case you get a pressure sore at some point.

Your insurance should also replace your hose and filters on a regular basis although possibly not as often as the mask. Be sure to have a backup hose.

Will I become dependent on, or addicted to, the CPAP?

No, the CPAP machine does not cause dependence and if your sleep apnea resolves because of weight loss, surgery, or any other reason, you will be able to discontinue the CPAP. But be sure the apnea is resolved by getting another sleep study.

On the other hand, though not dependence or addiction in a literal sense, some people become so used to the CPAP machine as part of their normal sleeping environment that it does take them awhile to get used to sleeping without it.

manometer and you should ask them to do this if you have any doubt. But, of course, that only means the pressure is correct at that time. A data download may also be reassuring. You may feel more reassured if you have the DME company disable the auto-off feature.

How do I clean the hose and mask and how often?

Your paperwork should give recommendations for cleaning your mask, hose and humidifier. Generally, they recommend a mild detergent followed by a thorough rinse. Sometimes vinegar is recommended but it is incompatible with some masks, so check the instructions, and be sure to rinse very well. **DO NOT** use bleach.

It is essential that your mask and hose dry completely every day after use, and after washing, to prevent the growth of mold and/or bacteria.

Your mask will absorb oils from your skin which will speed deterioration. It is amazing how bad some people let their masks get, both cleanliness and deterioration. You should wash your mask often enough to prevent this. This can vary from daily to once a week, depending upon the mask and your skin. There is a commercial mask cleaner and sanitizer machine available.

Is it really necessary to use distilled water in the humidifier?

All manufacturers recommend distilled water for the protection of the humidifier. If a significant portion of the water evaporates during the night, and you have relatively hard water, the deposited salts can have an insulating effect on the heating element and could potentially cause damage.

If you don't use the heat, have soft water, and most of it is left in the morning, then you **might** get away with tap water. Some people have certainly done this without problems. I cannot, however, recommend this.

Can I sleep on my stomach?

Yes, but there are two potential problems you might encounter, both concerning the mask. First, you might find that your mask is easily displaced when sleeping on your stomach. There are specially shaped pillows that may help with this.

Second, if you bury your face, and CPAP mask, in your pillow you might block the exhalation ports. Since you will still be getting plenty of air from the machine, you might not arouse immediately. But, with the ports blocked, you will be rebreathing your carbon dioxide which will probably result in headaches during the night or in the morning. This could be especially problematic if you have severe lung disease.

Talk to your doctor if you think this could be happening to you.

How long should it be before I can feel the difference?

That varies. Some people wake up after their first night on CPAP and say it was their best night of sleep ever. Other people take several weeks, or even months, before they really feel better. I had one gentleman who took an entire year to adapt to CPAP but he was determined.

Generally, the worse your AHI and/or desaturations, the more quickly you will feel the benefits. But if you have another significant sleep disorder, or other health problems, it may take a long time even with a high AHI.

If I lose weight will I be able to get off the CPAP?

Maybe. If you are significantly overweight, you should probably try to lose weight. It may or may not result in a "cure" for your sleep apnea but, regardless, in will probably result in better control of your apnea or a lower pressure requirement. And, of course, obesity is a significant health risk factor that should be addressed for reasons other than just sleep apnea.

As I discussed earlier, if you are young and have no anatomical anomalies such as a deviated septum, you have a better chance at resolving your apnea with weight loss. But there are no guarantees.

What should my "leak" numbers be?

That depends on the kind of machine you have. The leak is determined by measuring the amount of air moving through the machine. Some of that air is the normal airflow through the exhalation ports.

Some machines report the total airflow, some of which is normal. Other machines subtract the expected normal airflow through your mask and report the difference. That depends on the brand of machine you have.

A machine that does not include the exhalation airflow in the reported leak must have data on the model mask you use. If your mask is not in its database, either because your mask is a newer design or because you use a different brand of mask, your leak values will be erroneous.

All machines can tolerate a reasonable amount of leak and, for some machines, that is quite high. The bottom line is: read the manual for your CPAP machine and use the leak values as just one of several parameters in evaluating your progress.

Why does the machine continue to run even after I turn it off?

Some modern machines continue to run at a low level after

being "turned off" to dry the humidifier, mask and hose and to cool the motor. It should stop completely after a brief period.

Will sleep apnea make my insurance premiums go up?

Maybe. There are really two issues: medical insurance and life insurance.

With the recent changes in medical insurance, it is hard to predict how your premiums will be affected. It is possible that it may increase your premiums.

Life insurance is another matter. When applying for a new life insurance policy it is standard practice to review your medical history and, since sleep apnea is known to shorten life expectancy, it is possible that your premium will be affected. On the other hand, considering the prevalence of undiagnosed sleep apnea, if your apnea is adequately controlled with CPAP you may actually be at lower risk than someone among the general, untested population.

Will having sleep apnea affect my CDL?

The DOT is well aware of sleep apnea and the associated safety risks. The FAA and USCG are as well. They have published standards and requirements and your sleep doctor should be aware of these. The requirements have become rather onerous in recent years and, in my opinion, have become excessive and unreasonable. The doctor conducting your DOT, FAA or USCG medical exam will probably defer to your sleep doctor for clearance.

The DOT requires the doctor to screen for sleep apnea if your neck circumference is 17 inches or greater. Your insurance may require a home test which, as stated above, is NOT an appropriate screening test. The DOT will then require that your adherence (compliance) to the therapy be documented by a data download. The definition of adherence is, however, arbitrary and is not based on science. This is an example of uncontrolled bureaucracy but, unfortunately, it has to be dealt with.

Similarly, the USCG will require that you be retested without the CPAP every five years even if there is no reason to believe your apnea may have been resolved. This is a waste of your time and money but there is no option at this time. Unfortunately, for some people who have used CPAP for a long time may have a hard time sleeping without it. Also, as mentioned above, some people do not exhibit significant apnea for the first day or so after CPAP. This can make it challenging.

This means that you must be proactive. Be aware that, like many medical facilities, sleep labs often have a waiting list that may be weeks long. There will also be other delays in addition to the actual waiting list. Contact your medical examiner in advance to find out if you will need to have clearance from the sleep lab. If so, have him or her, or your family doctor, refer you to the sleep lab for reevaluation early.

Will my health insurance cover my CPAP machine?

Most insurance policies cover CPAP machines for diagnosed sleep apnea. They will have specific, published guidelines outlining the diagnostic requirements (lab accreditation, physician qualifications, etc.) and the severity thresholds required for coverage.

Many insurance companies follow the Medicare guidelines which, at the time of this writing, cover CPAP for AHIs above 15 and above and for AHIs between 5 and up to 15 if there are certain comorbidities such as: hypertension, heart failure, heart attack, stroke, hypersomnolence, and others.

A few medical insurance policies, especially those from businesses and agencies that "self insure", even if they have an insurance company administer the benefits, have had sleep apnea exclusions. I do not know whether this has changed under the 2009 US medical insurance law.

Is this sleep apnea thing a scam?

No. Diagnosis and treatment of sleep disorders in general, and sleep apnea in particular, has the potential of being one of the most cost effective of medical treatments.

In recent years there has been accumulating data linking sleep apnea, and other sleep disorders, with a number of medical/health conditions including hypertension, heart disease, obesity, and others. There is also data indicating that sleep apnea is vastly underdiagnosed. This has resulted in rapid growth of the field of sleep medicine. The "bean counters" at the insurance companies do not recognize this as the real drivers of the sleep field and assume the expansion is overuse or abuse.

Are there some practitioners that are working beyond their expertise for their own financial benefit? Sure. This happens in any rapidly growing field.

There are times that someone with mild sleep apnea meets the prescribing guidelines even though their apnea is not a major part of their sleep complaint nor are they at significant risk due to their apnea. Unfortunately, because of legal risks, these people are often pushed toward at least trying CPAP by their doctor. And every sleep specialist has had patients who surprised him or her with their improvement on CPAP.

But the treatment of sleep disorders, including sleep apnea, with scientifically verified therapy is a valuable and beneficial field of practice.

Having said all of that, back in the early 1990s I commented that obstructive sleep apnea was too big of a public health problem for the expensive product sleep labs delivered and predicted the rise of HST, which were already on the horizon. Considering the prevalence of uncomplicated obstructive sleep apnea in otherwise relatively healthy adults, and the improvement in auto-adjusting CPAP machines, I believe that CPAP should be available over-the-counter (OTC).

Can I adjust my CPAP pressure settings myself?

You can but, since your insurance company is "footing the bill", you probably should not at this time.

Although very rare, some patients will respond to CPAP therapy paradoxically. I have seen patients in the sleep lab simply stop breathing and precipitously desaturate when started on CPAP. Also, "blindly" changing your pressures may result in completely ineffective therapy.

Your doctor will use the data from your sleep study and from your machine download, his knowledge of your medical status, and his professional judgment in making any changes to your CPAP settings.

If CPAPs do become OTC, there will guidelines to help you select the best settings. The guidelines will also advise against those with certain medical conditions, such as severe lung disease or heart failure, using the OTC CPAP machines without medical guidance.

Chapter 11

Other treatments for sleep apnea

As discussed in Chapter 4, CPAP is the most commonly prescribed treatment for moderate to severe obstructive sleep apnea because it works, and it works consistently. Your doctor doesn't want to waste your time and his or hers on treatments that might or might not work.

CPAP is also often prescribed for mild sleep apnea, maybe even too often. But, again, this is because it consistently works and every sleep doctor has had patients with mild sleep apnea who amazed him or her with how well they did on the CPAP, and how much they improved.

As stated earlier, CPAP works consistently because it addresses the **mechanism** by which the apnea occurs, rather than the actual cause of the apnea. Nevertheless, there are alternatives to CPAP that sometimes cure the apnea and some that often bring improvement in the apnea and/or make the CPAP more tolerable. Let's discuss some of these now.

Other common treatments for sleep apnea include:

Oral appliances

Mouthpieces, often but not always fit by your dentist, are usually designed to reposition the lower jaw (mandible) and/or the tongue. They are often successful in reducing snoring and sometimes are effective in improving, or even fully controlling, sleep apnea. If your apnea is primarily driven by crowding by your mandible or your tongue then a device will possibly help.

Unfortunately, it can be difficult to determine who will benefit from an oral appliance. And, of course, the only sure way to know if it helped is to perform another sleep study adding to the expense. Many of the appliances are custom fit to the wearer, and therefore expensive, and for most people this requires purchase of the device before you can determine if it will be of benefit to you. There are adjustable devices that can be titrated in the sleep lab but are not widely used.

Are you a candidate for an oral appliance? Generally, you might benefit from an oral appliance if you fit more than one of these conditions:

> your apnea is mild to moderate
> you are not significantly overweight or obese
> your apnea occurs mostly while you are on your back
> your chin is not very prominent
> your tongue is not larger than average

Nose, Throat, and/or maxillofacial surgery

Several types of surgery may cure sleep apnea or, more commonly, simply make the CPAP more effective and/or more tolerable. We will cover a number of them later in this section but first let's discuss some general principles.

It is important to remember that obstructive sleep apnea is usually caused by a combination of multiple factors and is not just a mechanical "plumbing" problem. If it were just mechanical then the ENT surgeon would be able to cure it with a high degree of success.

If you are significantly overweight, your apnea is moderate to severe, you are middle aged or older, and you have no major anatomical abnormalities such as a severely deviated septum or a significantly recessed chin, then it is unlikely that ENT or facial surgery will correct your sleep apnea. It might, however, reduce the needed CPAP pressure and improve your comfort and tolerance, and this may be considered a success for the surgery.

But if you have mild apnea, are young, not overweight, have large tonsils and adenoids and/or a deviated septum, then there might be a good chance of a surgical cure for your apnea. Only your ENT doctor can assess the likelihood of surgical success in your case, and only after a thorough evaluation including a fiber-optic examination of the nasal passages and the pharynx.

There are no guarantees in life and, unless you have an unusually dramatic airway abnormality, the doctor will give you the assessment in terms of probability of success. Be sure to ask him or her what would constitute a successful surgery. And be wary if the doctor seems too sure of the chances for success.

Some of the common surgeries are:

Uvulopalatopharyngeoplasty, known as UPPP or UP3, consists of trimming the back edge of the soft palate, removing the uvula (the "hangy down thing"), and trimming soft tissue in the throat. It is very effective at controlling snoring, although the effect often diminishes in time (several years), but it is less effective at controlling sleep apnea. It has now become far less common than it was in the past.

> It is done under general anesthesia (they put you to sleep), usually in the hospital, and can be very painful. Although extremely rare, people have been known to die from postoperative complications which makes a hospital the preferred option. Sometimes people have trouble drinking, especially from a water fountain, after this surgery because the water, or other drink, comes out their nose.

Laser Assisted Uvulo-Pharyngeoplasty, or "LAUP" Is a multi-step procedure similar to the UPPP except it is done in a series of procedures, usually three to five, in the doctor's office. By doing it in smaller steps there is no need for general anesthesia. I do not know of anyone still doing this surgery.

> Many people say the pain is the same, just spread out over a longer period of time, and sometimes they don't complete all the phases because of this. Like the UPPP it is more effective on snoring than it is on apnea and the snoring often returns.

The "Pillar procedure", "Somnoplasty", etc, are proprietary surgical procedures, meaning that a company developed an instrument or device which they sell specifically for the procedure and the name is trademarked. Both of these procedures are more effective at controlling snoring than sleep apnea but in some cases of mild apnea, in a person who is not notably overweight, they may be sufficient.

> The "Pillar procedure" consists of inserting little nylon rods into the soft palate to provide stiffness and reduce the vibration. The rods are inserted through a needle and, because there is minimal cutting of the tissue, the pain is much less than with a UPPP or LAUP.

> "Somnoplasty" consists of inserting a small needle into the soft palate and using radiofrequency energy to cook the tissue in the palate. The resulting scarring stiffens the soft palate and reduces the vibration. Like the Pillar procedure, there is minimal cutting of the tissue.

Nose surgeries such as rhinoplasty, turbinectomy, etc., can be among the most successful of surgical remedies for sleep apnea. In cases of mild to moderate apnea in a person who is not overweight, nasal surgery may even cure the apnea. In other individuals the surgery may improve the apnea without curing it or reduce the CPAP pressure needed to control it.

> The nose is the narrowest part of the entire respiratory system. This means that correcting even a minor abnormality, such as a deviated septum or enlarged turbinates, can markedly reduce the resistance to airflow. A reduction in resistance means that less negative pressure is needed in the pharynx to pull adequate air through the nose. From my own personal experience, I would describe this surgery more as miserable than as painful.

Mandibular advancement, hyoid suspension, and tongue reduction are less common surgeries sometimes performed for sleep apnea.

A mandibular advancement consists of cutting the lower jaw (mandible) on both sides and advancing the chin slightly. Sometimes the upper jaw is also moved, making it a "maxillomandibular" advancement.

> Together with the base of the skull, the mandible makes a bony ring through which the anatomical structures of the neck must

pass. Since we all are normally born with the same structures, a smaller jawbone results in crowding of these structures. Expanding the mandible improves the situation and can reduce the apnea. It is probably less likely to be effective in those who are overweight or for those who already have a prominent jaw. Although it sounds very dramatic, those who have had both a mandibular advancement and a UPPP tell me it is less painful than the throat surgery.

A hyoid suspension anchors the hyoid bone to the thyroid cartilage. The hyoid is a small, free-floating, "U" shaped bone which serves as the attachment of some of the muscles of the neck and tongue. The theory is that by anchoring this bone there will be less tendency for the airway to collapse. It is effective in a percentage of people.

A tracheostomy is effective at controlling obstructive sleep apnea, and the only surgical treatment with a high degree of success in those who are obese. It consists of inserting a breathing tube into the trachea, the windpipe, which then opens at the base of the neck. The tube is capped during the day to allow normal speech. This is a dramatic treatment with a high complication rate and is only appropriate for sleep apnea in cases that are immediately life threatening.

Other Nasal treatments

Nasal treatments such as nasal sprays and drops or nasal expander strips can be quite beneficial. They are likely to control apnea, however, only in borderline cases.

"Borderline" in this case does not necessarily refer to a low apnea/hypopnea index. Instead it refers to the tendency for the airway to close off enough to be considered an apnea or hypopnea. As already discussed, a reduction of resistance in the nasal airway is effective because the nose is the highest resistance component of the respiratory system. Both nose sprays/drops and expander strips can reduce that resistance. The term borderline, in this case, refers to the negative pressure as near the threshold of airway collapse.

Nasal steroid sprays, either OTC or prescription, may help if nasal allergies are a problem. They do not have their maximum effect until they have been used for several days so they should be used regularly but prolonged use may not be indicated. Be sure to talk with your doctor about nasal steroids. Over-the-counter nasal decongestants, by contrast, have an immediate effect but can have a "rebound" where the congestion gets worse, leading to dependence. They are also contraindicated in people with high blood pressure.

Weight loss

Losing weight can be effective at improving or even curing sleep apnea. And virtually everyone who is overweight and has been diagnosed with obstructive sleep apnea has been told to lose weight. But most will agree that is easier said than done, and there is a reason for this.

The likelihood that weight loss will cure your sleep apnea depends upon a number of factors: level of obesity at the start and the amount of weight lost, age and tissue elasticity, other anatomical features such as a deviated nasal septum or hypognathia, etc.

> We have tested many, many people before gastric bypass surgery and after weight loss of 100 to 200 or more pounds. Generally, with no significant anatomical anomalies those under about 35 years of age often found their apnea dramatically improved or even cured. While those over about 50 often continued to have significant apnea but, fortunately, the apnea was often better controlled and with a lower CPAP pressure. (That's just a casual observation, not an epidemiological study.)

Weight loss strategies include:

Diet and exercise are the standard recommendation for weight loss and certainly the preferred approach most of the time. But research in the past few years has shown that the weight management pathways in your brain overlap with the sleep regulation pathways. This means that it can be very difficult to lose weight while your sleep is still disturbed by uncontrolled apnea and/or other associated sleep disorders. Fortunately, exercise itself can improve both your sleep and your sleep apnea.

Several medications for weight loss work by stimulating the "reward center" in your brain making you less inclined to seek food for such reward. This is the same way that smoking helps people lose weight. Some of these agents also act as stimulants and increase your activity levels. Other medication may affect the satiety center making you feel full sooner by a meal. Other medications help block the absorption of certain components of the diet, such as fat. These types of medications have problems of their own, for example: the "spotting" problem. Medication can be helpful in losing weight initially but the weight loss can be hard to maintain when the medication is discontinued, and unless you change eating habits, you will regain the weight.

Weight loss medications of the future will work on the body's energy balance system itself and, therefore, may affect sleep as well. In fact, sleeping medications currently in development may turn out to also help with weight loss.

Bariatric (weight loss) surgery can be effective for those who are very obese. There are several procedures that can be done from banding the stomach to a gastric bypass but none of them should be taken lightly. The amount of weight loss varies from person to person and can be in the hundreds of pounds but some individuals eventually regain much of the weight. Bariatric surgery may be the only realistic choice for someone who is massively obese.

> Weight loss is discussed in my ebook: **Lose Weight for your Sleep Apnea** available at Amazon. It needs updating which is forthcoming, so be sure to wait until it is noted as the Second Edition. A video version will be available at www.practicalhealthstrategies.com.

Positional training

Changing your sleeping position, usually to avoid sleeping on your back, can also be beneficial in some cases, but it is only rarely an effective treatment for adequate control of the apnea. If your initial sleep study indicated your apnea was primarily in only one position, most commonly on your back, this can be a reasonable therapeutic approach.

For many, but certainly not all, people the apnea/hypopnea index (AHI) varies significantly by position and for most of these it is worse when they on their back than when on their side. Some people are worse on their side.   But only a small percentage of people have an AHI on their back that is high enough to give them an overall diagnosis of sleep apnea while the AHI on their side is below the definition of sleep apnea (5.0 per hour).

> In years past we tried very hard to get these people to keep off their backs as the simplest therapy for their apnea. The standard recommendation was to put a tennis ball in a sock and sew it to the back of the pajamas. Unfortunately, it was not very effective because people would learn to pull their loose fitting pajama shirt around in their sleep to move the ball out from under them. There is at least one commercial product designed to help you keep off your back.

> So today, with more comfortable and tolerable masks and auto-adjusting CPAP machines, whenever someone has apnea only on his or her back, and it is severe enough to result in a significant overall AHI, we make the tennis ball suggestion but also treat the apnea with the more effective treatment: CPAP. We also make the tennis ball suggestion if the apnea is only on the back but not severe enough to give an overall AHI that qualifies as sleep apnea. In either case, we also recommend an ENT evaluation for any case of simple, positional sleep apnea.

Other lifestyle changes

Various behavioral changes such as avoiding alcohol and/or sedating medications and avoiding or quitting smoking are almost always recommended and sometimes can reduce the severity of the sleep apnea.

Alcohol and most sedating medications are respiratory depressants. That is, they reduce the drive to breathe. As obstructive sleep apnea is a multifactorial disorder, and respiratory control is a major factor, reducing the drive to breathe can increase the severity of the apnea.

Possibly just as importantly, alcohol and sedating medications reduce one's ability to arouse from sleep and it is the arousal that normally terminates the respiratory event. Thus, any sedating chemical including alcohol, sleeping medications, tranquilizers, or illicit "downers" will prolong the individual apnea or hypopnea. The prolongation of the respiratory events will often result in a greater oxygen desaturation.

The situation with smoking is more long term and, although you certainly should quit smoking, quitting has the effect of avoiding further damage more than of correcting prior damage. Smoking destroys tissue elasticity, effectively making you age faster. Thus, the effect of smoking on the apnea/hypopnea index is similar to getting older which is to increase the index. Additionally, the effect of smoking on the oxygen exchange function of the lungs will usually result in greater desaturation with each respiratory event.

Less common, controversial, and/or outmoded treatments include:

Music lessons and practice

Exercises for the muscles of the throat, such as singing and voice exercises or playing certain musical instruments, have been tried with some success. The idea is to strengthen and tone the muscles in the pharynx, but improved respiratory control may be just as important. The concept has been around for many years.

> Studies have looked at this approach, one using a musical instrument (probably any wind instrument would do) and one using exercises developed by a speech therapist. Both studies were limited to people with mild to moderate apnea, and both

excluded obese or severely obese people. And both mostly improved the apnea without actually curing it.

Although these studies are encouraging, there were some scientific limitations in the interpretation of them. Nevertheless, if you want to try this approach in addition to your CPAP, it probably will do no harm and may help.

NOTE: If you have high blood pressure or a heart condition, especially congestive heart failure, consult your doctor first.

Medication

Medication has been used in the past for the treatment of sleep apnea, but is rarely used today. The medications were either respiratory stimulants or REM sleep suppressants. Neither has been particularly successful.

Medications to stimulate respiration, either directly or indirectly have been used for both obstructive and central sleep apnea. They are helpful, especially for central apnea but they also have a tendency to disrupt the sleep.

Medications to reduce the amount of REM sleep have been used in treating obstructive sleep apnea. This is based upon the fact that obstructive apnea is often, although not always, worse in REM than in NREM. Implicit in this concept, however, is the assumption that REM does not serve an important function, which is certainly not true. The REM suppressants used were antidepressants.

Chapter 12

Glossary

AASM: American Academy of Sleep Medicine, probably the largest and most well established professional sleep organization, formerly the American Sleep Disorders Association (ASDA) and, before that, the Association of Sleep Disorders Centers (ASDC).

ABSM: American Board of Sleep Medicine, the credentialing body for doctors working in sleep medicine from the early 1990's until the early 2000's, an outgrowth of the original credentialing by the predecessors to the AASM. The ABSM continues to maintain its certification list but all new certification of doctors is done as a subspecialty their primary specialty.

ACP: abbreviation for Accredited Clinical Polysomnographer, the original doctorate level certification in sleep disorders.

ADAM Circuit: the original version of a "nasal pillow" style mask.

Adherence: the currently used term referring to CPAP usage; see Compliance.

Adjustment Insomnia: a subset of short-term insomnia under the new classification; it is an insomnia caused by an acute, external psychological stressor such as a loss or fear of a loss; also referred to as transient situational insomnia, the definition requires that it be of limited duration and specifically associated with the external stressor.

AHI: the "apnea/hypopnea index" expressed as the total number of apneae and hypopneae divided by the hours of sleep, necessary because the total number would differ after a long night of sleep and a short night of sleep, also helpful in determining if there is a positional or sleep stage component to the problem.

APAP: abbreviation for "Auto Positive Airway Pressure", see Auto CPAP below.

Apnea: to stop breathing or to not breathe. To be counted as an apnea for the purpose of diagnosing sleep apnea, the airflow signal must decrease by 90% or more and must be a minimum of ten (10) seconds in duration.

Apnea of Infancy: a common phenomenon of central apnea, observed in newborns, and reflective of an immature respiratory control system. Not usually pathological.

Arousal: a shift in the sleep EEG to a lighter level of sleep, used to refer to short duration shifts that do not last long enough to change the sleep staging.

Arrhythmia: lack of rhythm, used to refer to an abnormal pattern in the heart's electrical activity, the electrocardiogram (ECG or EKG).

Auto CPAP: a version of CPAP which adjusts the pressure to the current pressure needs. To do this it must increase pressure when respiratory events are detected and regularly test to determine if less pressure would be adequate. The reliability of the event detection is critical.

BiLevel PAP: a version of PAP that provides one level of pressure during inhalation and a lower level during exhalation (see IPAP and EPAP), especially useful in the treatment of hypoventilation; sometimes referred to as BPAP; also sometimes inappropriately referred to by the proprietary name "BiPAP" even when not referring to that specific brand of bilevel machine.

Cataplexy: a sudden loss of muscle tone while awake, commonly observed in narcolepsy, believed to be an intrusion of the muscle relaxation normally seen in REM sleep into wakefulness.

CBSM: Certified in Behavioral Sleep Medicine, a doctoral level certification in behavioral aspects of sleep, managed by the American Board of Sleep Medicine

Central apnea: an apnea in which there is no respiratory effort, no attempt to breathe.

Cheyne-Stokes respiration: a special subset of central apnea in which the airflow and respiratory effort wax and wane, the respiration gradually decreases until it stops and then gradually increases again to the normal level, often associated with heart failure.

Chin Strap: as the name implies, a strap under the chin to help hold the mouth closed and prevent mouthbreathing, can be as simple as a scarf but may be a specialized product from the medical equipment company.

Comorbidity: diseases, disorders and disabilities that coexist in a patient with the disease or disorder under discussion such as sleep apnea in this case.

Complex sleep apnea: a mixture of both central and obstructive sleep apnea syndromes, the technical definition requires that at least half of the respiratory events are central and that there are at least five central events per hour, often seen with the initiation of CPAP.

Compliance: the degree to which one uses the CPAP, usually now called Adherence; because of Medicare requirements, one is considered compliant with CPAP usage if they use the machine at least four (4) hours per day for seventy percent (70%) of the days during a thirty (30) day period. For Medicare purposes this thirty day period must be within the first ninety days. This definition of compliance was arbitrarily selected with no clinical research to support the specifics.

CPAP: Continuous Positive Airway Pressure, the most common version of PAP. In its simplest form the pressure is constant, except for the possible use of a ramp to start.

D,ABSM: a Diplomate of the ABSM, someone certified in sleep medicine by the ABSM.

Delta Sleep: The "deepest" stages of sleep characterized by slow waves called delta waves, the current scoring criteria call delta sleep "N3".

Desaturation: refers to a drop in the measured blood oxygen level during sleep. Oxygen levels during a sleep study are expressed as a percentage of the maximum carrying capacity (saturation) of the blood. This number should not be confused with a "blood gas" obtained by drawing arterial blood.

DIMS: abbreviation for Difficulty Initiating and Maintaining Sleep, used to group the various forms of insomnia in the very first classification of sleep disorders, now sometimes used as an abbreviation for insomnia.

DME: Durable Medical Equipment company, the usual supplier of PAP machines and supplies.

DPAP: Demand Positive Airway Pressure, a defunct version of PAP, last heard of in the 1990's, which tried to quickly increase the pressure to prevent respiratory events. The problem was that the rapid pressure increase would often awaken the user.

Dysrhythmia: an abnormal rhythm, used to refer to an abnormal pattern in the ECG or EKG.

ECG or EKG: the Electrocardiogram, the electrical activity of the heart normally recorded from the chest wall, the version using the letter K derives from the original German spelling and, when spoken, is easier to distinguish from EEG.

EDS: abbreviation for Excessive Daytime Somnolence (or Sleepiness), sleepy; the technical term used in sleep medicine is hypersomnolence.

EEG: abbreviation for Electroencephalogram, the "brainwaves".

EMG: the electromyogram, a recording of the electrical activity from muscles, an indication of the level of muscle tone or tension.

EPAP: Expiratory Positive Airway Pressure, refers to the pressure setting on a bilevel machine during exhalation.

EPR: Expiratory Pressure Relief, a proprietary name used by ResMed, a major CPAP manufacturer, for their version of expiratory relief.

Expiratory relief: a CPAP feature introduced early in this century which provides for a lower pressure during exhalation, it differs from bilevel PAP in that once the pressure is lowered it then returns to baseline gradually and without waiting for inhalation to begin.

Flex: a proprietary name used by Respironics, a major CPAP manufacturer, for the original version of expiratory relief.

Headgear: the harness, or occasionally cap, that is used to hold a CPAP mask in place.

Humidifier or Humidification: provides additional moisture to the CPAP air. There are two types of CPAP humidifier, a "cold passover" humidifier which is nothing more than a tank of water usually with air baffles and is rarely seen anymore, and a heated humidifier which is the modern standard. CPAP humidifiers moisturize the air in the CPAP circuit and should not be confused with a common room humidifier.

Hypersomnolence: sleepiness greater than the normally expected level, often abbreviated "EDS".

Hypertension: high blood pressure.

Hypervigilance: an increased or elevated level of alertness.

Hypnogogic Hallucinations: hallucinations occurring just prior to sleep onset, believed to be a symptom of a transition from wakefulness directly into REM sleep, a condition of being partially awake and partially in REM sleep, commonly associated with narcolepsy, but may be seen in any condition resulting is severe sleep deprivation or circadian rhythm disruption, such as shiftwork.

Hypopnea: a partial apnea. There are two technical definitions of hypopnea: (a) the airflow diminishes to 70% of baseline and the oximetry desaturates by 4 percentage points, the Medicare definition; or (b) the airflow diminishes to 70% of baseline with the oximetry desaturating by 3 percentage points. An hypopnea is detected by a different technology than an apnea.

Hypoventilation: breathing too shallow to provide for adequate gas exchange, generally documented by an accumulation of carbon dioxide in the blood, but may also result in a reduction of oxygen in the blood. The most common cause for this in the sleep lab is obesity.

Hypovigilance: a reduced level of alertness.

Inadequate Sleep Hygiene: a subset of chronic insomnia which is caused or exacerbated by a daily routine that is inconsistent with sleep onset and/or sleep maintenance; examples would include caffeine consumption late in the day, excessive alcohol consumption, random napping during the day or just prior to bedtime, insufficient daily activity, exercising just prior to bedtime, and others. There is sometimes a coexisting complaint of daytime sleepiness.

Insomnia: an inability to sleep. Although most doctors will simply use the general term insomnia, sleep specialists distinguish short-term and chronic insomnia and consider a number of different causes and patterns of insomnia.

IPAP: Inspiratory Positive Airway Pressure, refers to the pressure setting during inhalation on a bilevel machine.

K-complex: a specific brainwave pattern indicative of stage N2 sleep.

Macroglossia: a big tongue

Mask: the patient interface for the CPAP system, even though some examples would hardly be recognized as a "mask" by many people. New mask designs are introduced regularly, there are probably 30 or 40 available at any time; there should be one that is comfortable on your face.

Mixed apnea: an apnea which begins as a central apnea and ends as an obstructive apnea. Sometimes this occurs when the apnea sufferer hyperventilates (over breathes) after the apnea, blowing off CO_2, which causes a central apnea but when breathing effort resumes the airway collapses immediately and becomes obstructive. People with this pattern sometimes take longer to adapt to the CPAP.

MSLT: abbreviation for Multiple Sleep Latency Test. The test is used to quantify the level of sleepiness and consists of nap trials at two-hour intervals.

Mucosa: a moist lining tissue, the "skin" of the nose and mouth.

MWT: abbreviation for Maintenance of Wakefulness Test. This test is often used to quantify the level of sleep resistance for the purpose of clearing truckers, pilots, boat captains, etc., for their medical exam.

Narcolepsy: the classic disorder of "sleepiness" is really a disorder of sleep regulation. It is caused by an abnormality in the orexin/hypocretin system in the brain and can result in such symptoms as hypnogogic hallucinations, sleep paralysis, and cataplexy.

Nasal Pillows: small cushions that fit just into the nostrils to deliver PAP only into the nose; originally conceived to reduce mask bulk, this type of mask can also result in lower resistance and higher airflow

NREM or NREM Sleep: all stages of sleep other than REM sleep; further subdivided into stages, now referred to as N1, N2, and N3; accounts for about 75 to 80 percent of the sleep time for a healthy young adult.

Obstructive apnea (or hypopnea): a respiratory event which occurs because of a temporary obstruction of the airway in the area of the pharynx; the event must be a minimum of ten seconds in duration but can be much longer; to be considered an apnea, the airflow must decrease by 90% or more; to be considered an hypopnea, the airflow must decrease by 30% with a corresponding decrease in oxygen saturation (see Hypopnea definition for detail).

Obstructive Sleep Apnea Syndrome: a diagnosis indicating a minimum of five obstructive apneae and/or hypopneae per hour of sleep time, but often much worse; it has been associated with daytime sleepiness, memory and concentration difficulty, and with cardiovascular complications such as high blood pressure, heart failure, heart attack, and stroke. In children the definition is a minimum of one per hour.

Oximetry, Oximeter: the technology, and the machine, of blood oxygen measurement normally used in a sleep study, consists of a light beam passing through a thin area such as a finger or earlobe, measures the ratio of blood cells with oxygen and blood cells without oxygen, results expressed as a percentage of the total oxygen carrying capacity occupied.

Oxygen Saturation: the percentage of the total oxygen carrying capacity of the blood actually occupied by oxygen.

PAP: Positive Airway Pressure, a generic term for all the various versions of CPAP, Bilevel machines such as "BiPAP" and the specialized versions of noninvasive ventilation" not considered in this book.

Paradoxical Insomnia: a chronic insomnia presenting as a complaint of insomnia which cannot be objectively substantiated; formerly called "sleep state misperception" the sufferer sleeps by all objective measures, including EEG and observation by others, but complains of being awake much or all of the time period.

Periodic Limb Movements in Sleep (PLMS) or Periodic Limb Movement Disorder (PLMD): regular, rhythmic jerks or kicks of the legs (or arms) while asleep, specific scoring rules determine which leg (or arm) movements are counted, often confused with RLS by the general public and, sometimes, by physicians who are not sleep specialists. The diagnosis requires the movements cause a clinically significant sleep disturbance.

Pharynx: the connecting tube of soft tissue between the mouth and nasal passages at the upper end and the esophagus and trachea (windpipe) at the lower end, the part of the upper airway that both food and air must pass through; it is in this area that the obstruction occurs in obstructive sleep apnea syndrome.

Pickwickian Syndrome: named because of a character in Charles Dickens' "Pickwick Papers" and referring to the condition of having both obstructive sleep apnea and hypoventilation at the same time, the Pickwickian is significantly obese and notably hypersomnolent.

PSG or Polysomnogram: this is the basis of all laboratory based sleep studies. It consists of continuous recording of fifteen to twenty channels of physiologic data including EEG, eye movements, chin muscle tension, EKG, leg movements, airflow (using two different detection technologies), chest and abdominal breathing effort, and oximetry. The standard laboratory test must be monitored by a technologist present throughout the entire recording period.

Psychophysiological Insomnia: a specific subclassification of insomnia in which psychological arousal leads to physiological arousal which results in insomnia. Often initially associated with an external stressor, and therefore initially an adjustment insomnia, it becomes particularly challenging when the insomnia itself becomes the stressor which leads to the psychological arousal.

Pulse Ox: the oximeter.

Ramp: a comfort feature added to all modern CPAP machines, allows the machine to start at a lower pressure and gradually increase the pressure to the prescribed level, intended to help the user fall asleep.

RDI: the "respiratory disturbance index", often the same as the AHI, but may include RERAs in the count resulting in a higher value. Medicare and some insurance companies do not recognize RERAs and specify that only the AHI be used to qualify for CPAP.

REM or REM Sleep: Rapid Eye Movement sleep, also called Stage R, the stage in which most dreaming occurs, accounts for about 20 to 25 percent of the sleep time for a healthy young adult; important in the treatment of sleep apnea because the apnea often gets worse during this stage of sleep (the apnea may, however, be unchanged or, more rarely, even better during REM)

RERA: Respiratory Event Related Arousal, an EEG arousal associated with any scorable, or visible but unscorable, respiratory event, or snore; an unscorable event would include those events that would be scored as hypopneae except that the airflow or oxygen saturation did not decrease enough.

Respiratory Event: a generic term for any apnea or hypopnea, may be extended to include apparent decreases in airflow that are unscorable by the hypopnea definition because there is not sufficient desaturation or airflow decrease.

Restless Legs Syndrome (RLS): a phenomenon that occurs while awake, RLS consists of an irresistible urge to move the legs, interfering with sleep onset; symptoms occur when inactive and may occur at any time during the day but are often worse at night; often confused with PLMS which occurs during sleep and leads to sleep fragmentation and multiple awakenings

RPSGT: Registered Polysomnographic Technologist, the original credential for sleep techs performing and scoring sleep studies, managed by the Board of Registered Polysomnographic Technologists.

RST: Registered Sleep Technologist, a newer technologist credential managed by the American Board of Sleep Medicine.

Saturation: see Oxygen Saturation

Scoring: the process of analyzing a sleep study, usually performed by a registered technologist (RPSGT, RST, SDS), includes the sleep staging, counting of arousals, counting respiratory events, counting leg movements, notation of snoring, body position, movements and any unusual behavior; all of this data must adhere to specific scoring rules; although "computerized scoring" is available on most PSG systems, it is not considered acceptable and human scoring is required for accreditation of a sleep lab.

SDS: Sleep Disorder Specialist, another newer tech credential available only to respiratory therapists (registered or certified), managed by the National Board for Respiratory Care.

Shiftwork Sleep Disorder: sleep disturbance, whether manifesting as insomnia or hypersomnolence, due to any unusual work schedule, the most obvious being rotating shifts.

Sleep Disordered Breathing (SDB): refers to the entire range of sleep related breathing disorders including apnea, hypopnea, RERA, snoring, UARS, and hypoventilation.

Sleep Hygiene: refers to all the behaviors during the day and evening, and upon retiring to bed, that contribute to or detract from one's ability to fall asleep and/or stay asleep or obtain sleep of good quality. For example, drinking coffee just before bedtime would normally be considered poor sleep hygiene, whereas listening to soft music and light reading would be considered better sleep hygiene.

Sleep Paralysis: a condition in which a person is unable to move and becomes aware of this condition, thought to be a transition between wakefulness and Stage R (REM) sleep when muscle paralysis is normal, or vice versa; probably indicates a significant disruption of sleep regulation such as narcolepsy or shiftwork, or may indicate sleep deprivation.

Sleep Maintenance Insomnia: difficulty remaining asleep, a description of an insomnia complaint, not a diagnosis, may manifest as frequent brief awakenings or as more prolonged periods of wakefulness during the desired sleep period, may be abbreviated DMS for "difficulty maintaining sleep".

Sleep Onset Insomnia: difficulty falling asleep upon retiring, a description of an insomnia complaint, not a diagnosis, may be abbreviated DIS for "difficulty initiating sleep".

Sleep Phase Advance: a condition in which the biological clock component of sleep regulation has been shifted to an earlier time resulting in an early sleep onset and early awakening at the end of the sleep period. An example might be an elderly man who falls asleep in the early evening such as 7 pm and then awakens for the day at 3 am, after 8 hours, unable to return to sleep.

Sleep Phase Delay: a condition in which the biological clock component of sleep regulation has been shifted to a later time making it difficult to fall asleep at an earlier time if desired. An example would be a college student who has had only afternoon classes and studied late into the night all school year, which delayed the sleep phase, but then gets a summer job that starts at 5 am and needs to get to sleep early and arise early the next morning.

Sleep Spindle: a particular EEG pattern indicative of N2 sleep, a brief burst of brainwaves in a specific frequency range.

Sleep Stage: based upon the EEG, eye movements, and EMG; sleep is divided into four stages (N1, N2, N3, R).

Slow Wave Sleep: an alternative term for Delta Sleep, now called "N3".

Snoring: a rhythmic noise caused by the turbulent airflow and/or tissue vibration in the airway, mostly in the pharyngeal area. Snoring is NOT the same as sleep apnea but the factors contributing to snoring are many of the same factors that contribute to sleep apnea. Most, but not all, sleep apnea sufferers also snore. Many snorers also have sleep apnea.

Split-night: a combination sleep study in which the study is begun without CPAP (the diagnostic part) to document sleep apnea and then CPAP is instituted (the titration part) to determine the optimal CPAP pressure.

Staging: The process of reviewing the PSG to determine the sleep stage; part of the scoring process.

Titration: the incremental adjustment of one parameter to reach a measurable endpoint; in the case of CPAP, this refers to the incremental adjustment of the CPAP pressure to find a pressure that adequately controls the respiratory disturbance, minimizing the AHI preferably to below 5.0.

Turbinates: a fleshy structure in the upper nose; increases the surface area of the nasal mucosa to increase the ability of the nose to warm and humidify the air before it reaches the lungs.

UARS: Upper Airway Resistance Syndrome, used to describe the sleep disturbance caused by airway resistance which does not rise to the level of causing an apnea or hypopnea.

Appendix I: Some Sleep Hygiene Tips

The following tips have been found to work for many people who have trouble sleeping.

Personal habits:

Try to establish a routine that allows you go to bed and get up at approximately the same time every day. This will help strengthen your biological clock and put your body into a good "sleep-wake rhythm". Of course, this can be difficult or impossible if you are a shiftworker or work an unusual schedule.

Regular exercise can help deepen your sleep. It should be moderate and invigorating but not exhausting (unless you are an athlete in training).   However, exercise shortly before bedtime may prevent you from falling asleep.

For several hours before bedtime, avoid alcohol; beverages with caffeine; chocolate; heavy, spicy, sugary or sugar-filled foods; and smoking. They can affect your ability to fall asleep or reach deep sleep.

Limit fluid intake before bedtime to help reduce nighttime urination.

Sleep environment:

If your bedroom is too cold or too hot, it can keep you awake. Find a comfortable temperature setting for sleeping (most people sleep better with a slightly lower room temperature), and keep the room well ventilated.

Block out all distracting noise; a "white noise" source is OK. Eliminate as much light as possible, but total darkness is not necessary. Just enough light to prevent tripping if you need to visit the bathroom is OK and avoid turning on the bathroom light. A motion sensitive nightlight may be helpful.

Bedding that is uncomfortable can prevent restful sleep. This can include too soft or too hard of a mattress, dirty bed linens, too thick or too thin pillow, bedbugs, etc.   Evaluate whether or not this is a source of your problem, and make appropriate changes. (Mattress firmness, pillow thickness, etc., are personal preferences.)

Use your bed for sleep and not as an office or recreation room. Don't watch TV or read for extended periods in bed; a few minutes is OK. Don't study, pay bills, or other tasks that require concentration in bed. Your brain should "know" that the bed is for sleeping.

Pre-sleep routine:

A regular presleep routine such as a warm bath or a few minutes of reading can help your brain know it's time to shut down and go to sleep.

Leave your worries about job or family for another time. It may help to have a "worry pad" on your nightstand to write down any last minute thoughts and save them for the next day.

Relaxation techniques before retiring may relieve anxiety and reduce muscle tension.

Get into comfortable sleeping position. If you don't fall asleep quickly do not allow yourself to get frustrated, this will only arouse you more and make sleep more difficult.

If you find yourself getting frustrated, get up and move to another room with soft lighting and read until you become sleepy. Avoid the TV or computer (including tablets or phones).

Some foods such as milk or bananas may help you sleep.

Other Factors:

Physical symptoms associated with several medical conditions are known to inhibit or disrupt sleep. Common examples include arthritis, heartburn, menstruation, headache, hot flashes; talk to your doctor about controlling these symptoms.

Sleeping difficulties are also associated with psychological factors such as anxiety, depression, grief, and stress. Your sleep doctor can help you determine the problem and the best treatment approach for you. Sleeping medications may be appropriate for short term use.

Many prescription and over-the-counter medications, and dietary supplements, can cause sleeplessness as a side effect. Ask your doctor or pharmacist if this is a possibility with your medications or supplements.

Sleep medications may distort the organization of your sleep and treat the symptoms of insomnia without correcting the underlying problem. The result can be less than fully restful sleep and your goal should be to rediscover how to sleep naturally.

These tips will help many individuals but not everyone. If you still have difficulty sleeping after following these suggestions, speak with your sleep doctor. Also see programs available at www.practicalhealthstrategies.com including an online insomnia video program: "How to Conquer Your Insomnia".

Appendix II: A screening questionnaire we sometimes use

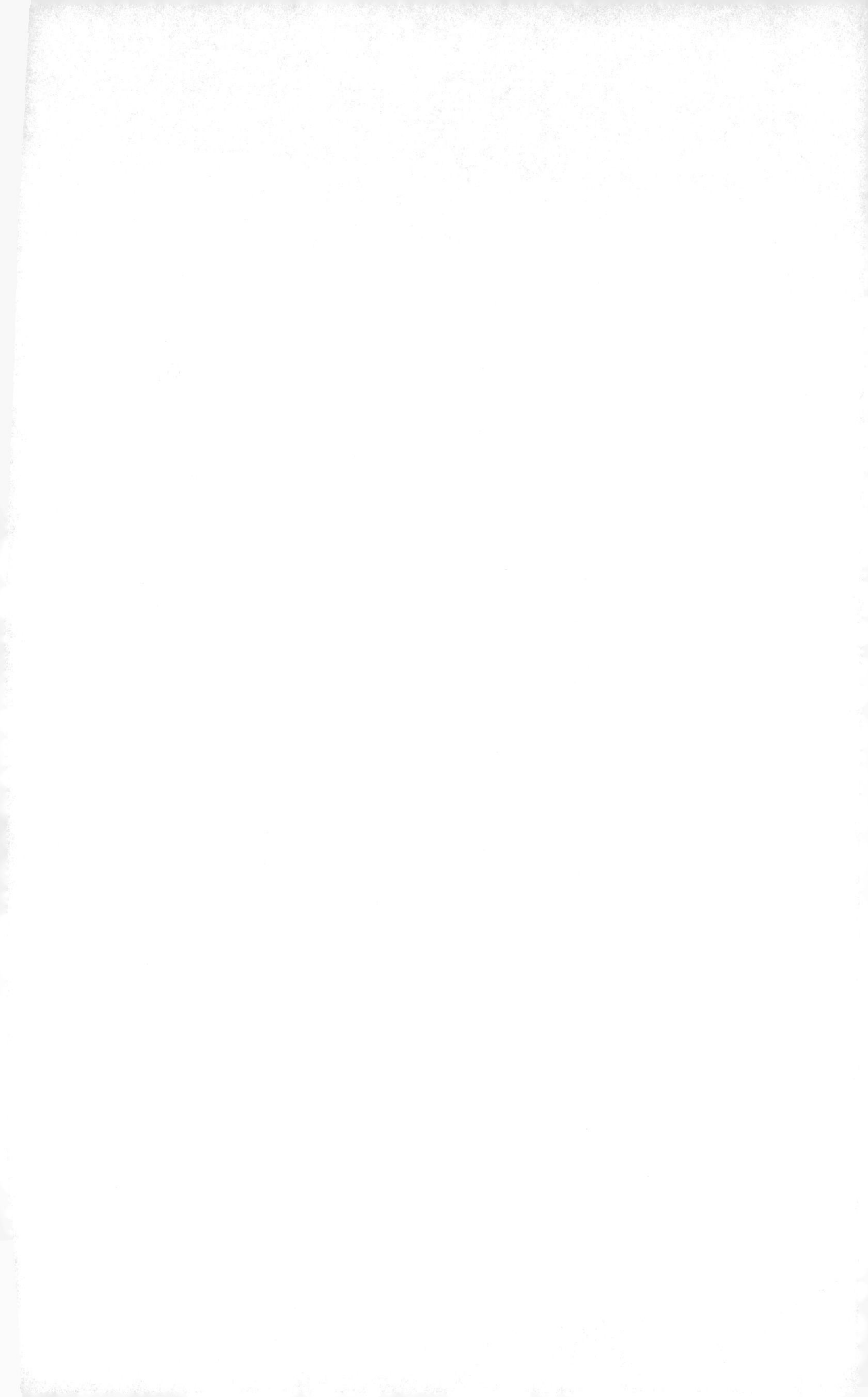